The Human Restoration Project

Restoring Health and Resiliency in the Chaos of the Modern World

MARE TOMASKI

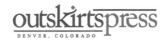

The opinions expressed in this manuscript are solely the opinions of the author and do not represent the opinions or thoughts of the publisher. The author has represented and warranted full ownership and/or legal right to publish all the materials in this book.

The Human Restoration Project
Restoring Health and Resiliency in the Chaos of the Modern World
All Rights Reserved.
Copyright © 2014 Mare Tomaski
v4.0

Cover Photo © 2014 thinkstockphotos.com. All rights reserved - used with permission.

This book may not be reproduced, transmitted, or stored in whole or in part by any means, including graphic, electronic, or mechanical without the express written consent of the publisher except in the case of brief quotations embodied in critical articles and reviews.

Outskirts Press, Inc.
http://www.outskirtspress.com

ISBN: 978-1-4787-2760-6

Outskirts Press and the "OP" logo are trademarks belonging to Outskirts Press, Inc.

PRINTED IN THE UNITED STATES OF AMERICA

Acknowledgements and Gratitude

Our lives are woven in a giant tapestry of fellow seekers on the paths throughout life, and the people upon my life-walk are many and varied. They are friends who have indulged me over the years when I came across some new bit of information, or a class or book that had me jazzed up about some new topic. Without these beloved companions my life would not be as rich. Jimmy, Rachel, Ben, Robin, Julia, Jillian, Nikki, Diane, Sahar and Jeanne my love to you all for your friendship and support. To "The Goddesses" for years of inspiration and love–you fabulous women rock my world! Many thanks go to those friends who read through a chapter or two and offered their sage advice: Dan Lewis, Michael Delman, Karen Bird, Jillian Dickert, Mike Fritz, Kym Croft Miller and Pamela Langley thank you for your feedback and friendship. My love to all my sweet friends at The Peace Abbey for creating a space where hearts can always rest. To my musical comrades, you make everything sparkle, thank you for helping me grow and for your beautiful music.

To my colleagues in the alternative health field, my admiration and respect for loving the world and wanting healing and happiness for all. To Jane Bowler my sister in all things fabulous, I'm so glad you are in my life. To my students and clients who have honored me beyond words by trusting me with your bodies, hearts and minds for all these years—thank you from the bottom of my heart. To my teachers who set me on this path and guided me with wisdom and love, I am most grateful. To my fabulous editor Maura Norton thank you for your swift responses and helping to make the words flow. To Rhiannon and Paloma, my sweet girls. Many thanks to my mom and dad who instilled a love of books in me at a young age and to my uncle Jude for your kind heart and supportive words. To all The Ancestors and The Grandmothers—wela'lieg for guiding me and watching over me. My gratitude for this big, beautiful, messy world within which we live, I bow down in deep reverence and awe.

"But the times are changing, and the indications are many that this civilization has begun to pass from the age of pure materialism to a desire for the realities and truths of the universe."

—*Edward Bach*

Contents

Introduction 1
The Quest to Find Inherent Health (or "my story") 6
The Disease Cycle 19
The Placebo Effect and the Power of the Mind to Heal ... 35
Free Will 44
Nourishment (also known as "diet") 54
The Truth About Sugar 67
Movement and Posture 73
Touch the Earth 84
Listening to the Body 97
Going Unplugged 106
Not Good Enough 118
Resiliency and Accepting What Is 132
The Art of Living 142
Meditation and Stillness 149
The Medicine of the Future 167

Introduction

Over decades of trial and error I have restored a host of deficiencies that had been lost in the early parts of my life. This journey was nurtured and fed by simple truths that have stood the test of time and remain part of a foundation of health and well being I've come to expect. These principles have now become increasingly accepted within a wider world view as it seems our culture has matured beyond the "tree hugging, granola-eating hippie" stigma, thank goodness. All those tree huggers were onto something and science is proving just what traditional cultures and our grandmothers and great-grandmothers knew: stick with the earth and you can thrive. I hope to do my part to herald these practices as not just a good idea but as vital medicine for a weary world.

I didn't acquire this information from my doctors. I didn't learn this information in school or church or girl scouts or gym class. In other words, these are not things that were a part of normal everyday life as a child growing up in North America.

Restoring health and well being was not only about the absence of physical disease, although that was part of it. I was also hoping to create or uncover, an internal feeling of ease, happiness, strength and stability that went beyond just the absence of illness. I was seeking an overall vitality with an intuitive knowing about how to take mindful and balanced care of my life amid all the conflicting information out there. What I wanted was to take charge of my own health, my own life, and to develop my "Inner Physician," as time and again conventional medicine was not all that adept at resolving many things that troubled me. It was a process of restoring an original state of vibrancy that had become mired with the wounds of life, fears, poor lifestyle habits and self limiting beliefs. Health was still there, it was buried, but still it was there. It took some time to feel like I was communing with health again and it is an ongoing project but I've come a long way upon the road. Now I can look back and say, it was and is my mission in life. The Human Restoration Project is a journey any one can embark upon, you must find your own way but I hope within these pages you will find inspiration and an outline to follow as you start, or continue your own Human Restoration Project.

There are a host of life-affirming choices we can make that have stood the test of science and time. We've all heard them by now and somewhere inside we all know they are essential keys to health: a whole-food diet rich in local organic vegetables and fruits, regular exercise, a positive mental/emotional outlook, meaningful work, and the ability to cope with and manage stress in a sustainable way. These are just five of the basics that have many tributaries running off them. We can probably all agree that these five principles are ones to implement consistently over the long haul and we can be confident that these principles have been a restorative force for hundreds of years even as countless fads have come and gone.

First Steps on the Path

While growing up it seemed to me that the normal and accepted way to eat was a steady consumption of packaged food-like substances along

INTRODUCTION

with other marginally acceptable food choices, and far too much sugar and alcohol. I was also constantly observing extreme hyper-vigilance, tight and painful muscles and joints, over-active minds, not enough bodily activity or sleep, and the inevitable downward slide into illness, aging and eventual death, all being labeled as "normal." I noticed both for myself and others, that a suppression of authentic emotion and vulnerability (improperly known as "weakness") was also considered normal. The whole person on so many levels was a jumbled bag of discomfort and pain physically, mentally, emotionally and existentially. A depleted and weary existence seemed like some kind of cultural badge of honor. It meant you were working hard and sacrificing yourself for something. I simply could not, and still cannot accept that the potentially exquisite human experience could be reduced to this. It seemed equally unacceptable to have some collective agreement that this was a "normal" way to live.

Of course I cannot throw a blanket over everyone and say this stressed out, hyper-vigilance and tension is a universal condition. There are certainly people living contented, well-balanced lives with high levels of self respect, internal ease and good health. Plenty of people grow up in loving families, are taught self respect, and are shown how to live a basically balanced and self-determined lifestyle. Not to mention that some level of angst and struggle is part of being alive, and I am in no way suggesting we need to abolish adversity to be healthy and happy. In fact a lot of growth happens during those times of struggle, especially if you have acquired tools for managing stressful and difficult periods in life. Even those well adjusted folks may at some point in their lives experience short term, situational periods of unrest, poor health, depression and anxiety. The resilient person can adapt and navigate during those inevitable times. Resiliency has its own chapter here and is a pillar of The Human Restoration Project. Developing the virtue of resiliency in our lives can reveal the inherent power and strength of our potential as human beings. There is something inspiring and uplifting about witnessing a resilient person in action. Some where inside we all know we posses this trait, and in the presence of resiliency depression and anxiety can be eased.

Add to the inevitable ups and downs of life our all-consuming and intrusive media presence, the internet, constant phone connection and social media updates, and we are sure to live with plenty of over stimulation and bad news to amp up our stress response. We live with all of those distractions now, high levels of chaos are part of the world we now find ourselves living in, and few are immune to the effects of this current model of culture. How can we adapt and manage what we have become? It may seem daunting but there are plenty of common sense lifestyle choices we can make every day to encourage some level of peace and sanity. First we must restore, build up reserves and let go of the idea that it is normal to be so depleted and worn out. Taking care of ourselves must be moved to the top of the priority list and we need to learn just how to make that a reality.

There have been some well researched studies on longevity and adaptability among people who live to be one hundred years and older with a variety of life experiences. There have also been some amazing reports of people who have endured war, torture, abuse, and even the Holocaust who then went on to live well-adjusted lives well into their eighties, nineties and beyond. I find their tales fascinating and informative and have taken to heart some of the things that yield positive results from those stories. It appears clear to me that there are themes and consistent qualities and traits that run through these stories of triumph over adversity. These themes can inform us in our quest for health and longevity, themes like: personal responsibility, self respecting choices, staying informed, honest self inquiry, neutral listening and the ability to forgive both ourselves and others that become the foundation of a life well lived, amidst a variety of life experience. There are no one-size-fits-all instructions when it comes to navigating the choppy waters of life, and this book is not an instruction manual. The Human Restoration Project is an invitation to consider for yourself that you have more influence over your health than you may have been led to believe. We have more information now than ever before to help us along the way. The only catch is, we cannot have someone else develop

INTRODUCTION

these attitudes and habits for us, and there is no pill that will magically take away our suffering. We've tried that route and it has largely failed too many people with a myriad of unsavory side effects and drug interactions that cause worse problems than the original illness and in some cases, even premature death.

An Inside Job

You can cultivate the strength, resiliency, and self respect to weather the storm—but it's an inside job. Our strength comes from the inherent human powers we all possess, not from an outside source. The doctor, the medications, the psychologist, the self-help books, friends and family provide important support systems and may help take the edge off, or alleviate symptoms for a time. Yet there is a stronger healing force far greater than these outside influences, that would like to conspire with you to magnify from within, that which is reaching for health and well-being. The question is, how do we connect with and awaken that force? How can we maintain steady interaction and communication with it? I hope after reading further here you will come away with a renewed sense of inspiration to find for yourself the magnificent healing potential we human beings have been endowed with. I hope you will feel ready and excited to shift into consistent health enhancing lifestyle choices, turn on the forces of innate healing given to you at your creation and share them freely and joyfully with the people in your life. So let us begin The Human Restoration Project.

To our collective health!
Mare Tomaski
Boston Massachusetts
April 2013

The Quest to Find Inherent Health (or "my story")

This desire to be at ease and healthy was stirred somewhere in my mid-teens and has continued over the past thirty years or so. My yearning for well-being felt a bit like a quest. Like some long search for the Holy Grail of Authentic Health that at times eluded me for years. Maintaining the health and resiliency I've created has become a solid way of life, and sharing what I've learned has become a passionate part of my career as an alternative health practitioner. This is not to say I don't still have remnants of old patterns that show up on occasion or relationships that have run amok and not been repaired, and I still have times that I don't make the healthiest choices or move my body as often as I'd like. The difference now is that these things are not catastrophes that affect my health and contentment. I now make more consistent, uplifting and self-respecting choices and the unhealed places have shrunk down to a manageable scale. Life is about relativity to me now and ideas of right or wrong have been replaced by shades of gray. The experience of being alive has become a bit of an experiment where the defining lines between absolutes are bit blurred. There are principles of universal law, of this we can be sure. Like gravity, and like days turning to nights, and that we live upon a planet that can only absorb the folly of humans so much before things become out of balance. That sky, water, and soil require our respect and care. That the earth and the people inhabiting earth are our treasures, while greed and materialism tend to offend those laws. Of those universal laws we can be sure. How we abide in those laws is personal choice. Each one of us will find what brings meaning to us in our own way. So this is not a specific instruction manual but more of an idea sharing project. I'd like to share some of the strategies I used to achieve my health and happiness goals here with you. Incorporate what makes sense to you, perhaps consider thinking about what challenges you and leave what ever doesn't make sense to you aside.

The Long and Winding Road to Clarity

I grew up on the northeast coast of New England where our ongoing imprint, if you will, is one of hard work, harsh judgments and high intellectualism. Cold weather, and a long standing legacy of puritanical influence spanning hundreds of years have left their mark. We are a tough breed, and I've spent a lot of time observing the particular mindset and lifestyle of people living in a cold, and sometimes harsh environment. I've spent even more time trying to neutralize those hard edges from my own personality. In many ways I admire our regional personality here in the Northeast. We are a product of our land and climate to which we have adapted with the best of our abilities. We are products of the indelible history of revolution and we pride ourselves on education, hard work, and our deeply stoic attitudes. We are both conservative and progressive and although I could not leave here soon enough as a young adult for the wide open spaces of the west, I am most happy to be here now. Attitudes are expanding and while people have typically been wonderfully loyal and solid here in this place where things like to stay the same, I am now seeing an additional open minded acceptance of new ideas that has come to roost here in the past fifteen years or so.

While most of my professional experience has its roots in good old stoic New England, it does seem like no matter where I find myself, there are people who have an internal angst of their very own to grapple with. We could say that regionally, countries, states, cities, and towns all take on their own specific personality based upon their history, climate, and social structures. Much of what I've observed has been not only through my private wellness practice but also through travels and taking countless classes all over the United States, South and Central America, and parts of Europe. People are people, and we all struggle with many of the same challenges when it comes to *Life, Liberty and the Pursuit of Happiness.*

A large part of finding inner happiness for me, was to cease resisting the parts of myself that I had sent into exile. The craggy rocks of my tough love upbringing that I tried to kill, had to find a place back into my heart before I could allow them to melt a bit. Sending them away to some dark corner of my mind was doing far more harm than good. A place for each dimension of human-ness needs to be carved into our acceptance, even the stuff lurking in the shadows; the self-loathing, guilt, and shame. We all have those parts to ourselves, so we might as well accept them. There will be people and situations that activate those past memories. Know that it always takes two people to create a disturbance. If someone does not take responsibility for their part, all you can do is own your part and move on. With some level of surrender to every part of ourselves, the practice of life-supporting choices can become far stronger than the self-destructive forces in our lives. Set your compass to those life-affirming principles before making choices. Ask yourself: does this choice support and encourage life or does it support and encourage decay? I will refer to those two questions often here and encourage you to ask them of yourself.

Do your choices create health in your body, mind, and spirit, or do they create disease and decay?

Picking Up Steam

After high school I began to take classes and read every book I could get my hands on about nutrition, Chinese medicine, yoga, homeopathy, naturopathy, herbs, internal cleansing diets, fasting, juicing, and exercise. By this time I knew college was not for me, so I plunged into alternative culture with both feet and felt I had finally found a place that was full of insight, common sense, and some answers to my questions. Those were some of the most invigorating days of my young life. I met some wonderfully creative people who were inspired and committed to exploring the timeless wisdom of other cultures and other realities in regards to what might be the right way to live. After all, that was what I wanted to know; what is the right way to live? It would take years to realize that there isn't one right way to live, yet I am grateful the question drove me to at least try to find out. I did discover some general themes to work within that do not offend natural law, and those are the things that inform my choices now. Nothing trumps natural law—nothing. Offend it at your own peril and be ready to accept the consequences if you make those choices; natural law abides in one primary principle and that is to support living systems in their continued existence.

Learning to respect and understand natural law is a worthy endeavor if you want to restore—and then thrive.

All of my explorations into that which supports life added value and helped me circle the wagons around core themes that held strong amid a swirl of passing fads and trends that did not hold up to the test of self-experimentation, science, and time. A passionate interest in traditional systems was driven from somewhere inside, some inner knowing that was pointing in the direction of truth even though it was often going against the culture of those times. I grew up in the '70s and the norm of that era was Wonder Bread, Kraft macaroni and cheese, Spam, Chef Boyardee, and lots and lots of television. My mom and grandmothers cooked great meals for us which was a wonderful thing even though what my taste buds got quickly and powerfully used to was artificial flavor, fat, sugar, and salt. Thank goodness for those home cooked meals in between all the junk food habits. The cultural trends of those years did not let go of me easily, it took years to replace those alluring but destructive tendencies.

As I got closer to my true north, well, I traveled west. The desire for adventure became part of the impetus that drew me to the high desert of northern New Mexico in 1994. New Mexico is a nearly perfect place to immerse into alternative healing, and I chose to start my formal education by enrolling in a two year program in massage therapy at the New Mexico Academy of Healing Arts in Santa Fe. It was the most enjoyable school experience I've ever had. I absorbed everything massage school and the Southwest had to offer. I found pieces of myself slowly beginning to sneak a peek at new possibilities for expression.

Back in my late teens and early twenties I did not consciously know that so many of my fellow humans were, like me, enduring lives of such quiet desperation, but I considered that maybe I wasn't completely alone in this. With time and a good dose of inner work, I came to see I most certainly was not alone in these tension patterns and feelings of weariness. Different people feel it in varying degrees and I felt it like a freight train at times. I realized that for probably my entire life part of my tension and sadness was not only my own inner turmoil but the subtle and constant sense of absorbing the suffering of the world. How could I live in this world with all this suffering? Should I try to shut down? Toughen up? Tune out? Why did I have to be so sensitive? Most of the time it was nothing but trouble to be this sensitive. It downright tired me out. I wondered how on earth would I ever manage.

Know Thyself

To be a sensitive soul in this hard-edged world can be perilous for the central nervous system, and the sooner the sensitive person accepts and respects this genetic endowment the better life will be for them. If you are a sensitive soul, take heart. There is now quite a bit of discussion and support out there for the twenty percent of us born with nervous systems that process deeper, faster, and more complex bits of information. "The Highly Sensitive Person" has now been recognized as a genetic sub group of people, and we now know that sensitivity is not a choice, nor is it a flaw. Highly Sensitive People are often exceptionally creative and diligent workers and attentive, thoughtful partners. They are often times intellectually gifted and keenly intuitive individuals. We can turn to the research and support of Dr. Elaine Aron and countless others, who have identified The Highly Sensitive Person.[1] Dr. Aron believes, Highly Sensitive People could contribute much more to society if this inherent trait was understood and honored more fully. There are biological reasons for sensitivity, such as a hyper responsive amygdala, the brain center that assesses threats and processes emotional stimulation. Research suggests that sensitivity could also be linked to variations in gene expression in the nervous system, notably genes related to production of the neurotransmitters serotonin and dopamine. During every day tasks the nervous system of the sensitive person experiences less latent inhibition, they absorb and detect even the most subtle of incoming stimulus and more of their brains are highly activated from moment to moment. Andrea Bartz, a Brooklyn based writer and editor, explained this level of sensitivity eloquently in the July/ 2011 issue of Psychology Today Magazine:

> *Settling into a chair for coffee with a friend, Jodi feels her heart begin to pound. Tension creeps through her rib cage. Anger vibrates in her solar plexus. But she's not upset about anything. The person across from her is. Jodi soaks up others' moods like a sponge.*

---

[1] Aron, E., The clinical implications of Jung's concept of sensitiveness, *Journal of Jungian Theory and Practice, 8, 11-43.*

On a walk through her neighborhood in Ottawa, Canada, her attention zeroes in on the one budded leaf that hasn't unfurled; it brings a lump to her throat. The cawing of a far-off crow galvanizes her attention. An abandoned nest half-hidden amid the treetops fills her with awe.

Absorbing the emotions of others from a mile away, and noticing the beauty of that one unfurled bud on a tree could slay me in an instant. My sensitivity perplexed me for years and I am so grateful there is discussion and support around high sensitivity out there now. Discovering the facts about my physiology was one of several enlightening realizations that changed my life immeasurably and I am now very aware of not disregarding my sensitivity. Instead, I allow it to be a guiding force, and I have come to appreciate being sensitive as one of my greatest assets as an alternative health care practitioner, writer, and musician.

The suggestions in this book are for anyone living with more stress than they care to, which seems to be most of us. However, for the sensitive person the ideas put forth here are essential. The sensitive person must understand and respect the intensity of feeling when they are overwhelmed by taking some quiet time. Eating right and managing stress in mindful ways is also imperative. Engaging in work that allows creativity is extremely important, and despite the cultural admiration of going through life at hyper speed the sensitive person must take time every day to rest their senses, or they will quickly burn out. Nurturing a sense of calm is not weakness, especially considering the sensitive among us take in more information than the average person. The cellular receptor sites of sensitive people are more innervated, so physiologically we feel everything more acutely. For all of us, no matter what our threshold, over stimulation of the nervous system leads to physical exhaustion, anxiety, depression and fatigue. The strategies within these pages will, if done consistently, teach you how to manage stress in sustainable ways regardless of your inherent constitution. We are all made of basically the same stuff, the central nervous system was designed to thrive if we do not offend its inherent intelligence. Modern life, quite frankly, is a major offender of our ages old operating system.

Lifelong Learning

After years of study, and idealizing my teachers, little did I know there would come a time when information would start to spring from within me, not from a book or a class but from somewhere inside. We all have the capacity to develop this intuition through deep listening to our subtle thoughts and ideas and through raising our consciousness with health enhancing lifestyle choices. One of the first moments this piercing clarity occurred was while I was living in New Mexico. I was driving north on the Old Taos Highway, which leads up a massive hill near the Rio Grande Gorge. The hill is so high I thought I would drive right off the edge of it. The gorge is a massive ecological wonder, an epic slice right through the earth. The sky was getting closer and the gorge was getting wider, and I thought I might be swallowed up whole. A moment of fear in my belly gave way to feeling totally perceptive and quite content with the idea of being swallowed whole by the earth. I was so grateful for the beauty of the Southwest and felt a strong sense of equilibrium and what I might call a *right-ness* about everything in that moment. Everything was shimmering; I felt the tension drain away from my face, and my shoulders relaxed. My whole body began to surrender, time slowed down, and some kind of wider perception began to emerge. The enormity of the sky above and the massive chasm of the Rio Grande Gorge delivered a clear message about the opposing forces of fear and joy. In an instant, the weight of worldly suffering juxtaposed with my sudden feelings of relaxation and joy hit me in a conscious way. There is a way to manage life, I thought, it is about seeing it all, the dark and the light *without resistance.* The dark and the light go together. The dark makes the light that much sweeter. To resist this is futile. It was about gaining higher perspective and letting go physically, which I was feeling as I inched closer to the top of the hill. Talk about higher perspective! I began to laugh and cry at the same time. Laughing because I was so blessed to be having this incredible moment with the earth and crying for about a hundred reasons I could barely grasp, even while understanding them with a much fuller perspective. How can so much beauty also contain so much pain and sorrow? How can we be given this incredible planet and these incredible bodies and yet be so very careless and destructive with them? Why can we not respect and protect this precious earth and ourselves? Right there and then after the smallest glimpse of total harmony, I had a momentary peek into it all being somehow the biggest lesson of being here, of what it means to be a person living upon this earth. Surrender, acceptance and showing up to do my part seemed to be the cure. It was a fleeting moment of clarity, and although it didn't last, and fear would come back again, it altered me inside. Did the altitude alter my attitude? Was it the hugeness of the sky or the depth of the gorge that blew my heart and mind wide open? I still do not really know but it didn't matter. I made a promise to the big blue New Mexico sky that if I could free myself and live with more relaxation and acceptance, I would do my part to help other people gain some of their own freedom and happiness. It was a promise to myself and to whatever powers were out there as I continued to reflect on all the human pain and suffering contrasted against the enormity of the New Mexico sky, the Rio Grande Gorge and my expanded awareness. To this day, relaxing my body, paying attention to the earth and feeling, I mean *really feeling* the gift that was given to us with this gorgeous floating planet we live upon re-inspires me and shows me the way to inner peace almost without fail. There was way more to inspiration than I understood. Relaxation became a huge importance to me. I had not known how amazing it felt to be soft and surrendered and after that experience I began to see tension in the people around me more clearly and some times the way to help would just appear, seemingly out of "no where"—but clearly the cure came from inside. It came from the place inside all of us that maintains the health that cannot be taken away from us. It may get covered over with pain, betrayal, and loss but that constitutional health remains there, deep inside of each one of us, just waiting for us to relax enough to unleash it.

After moving back to New England about a year later, I would spend the next decade absorbing the beauty of this truth and allowing it to spread out over all my cells, slowly replacing the negativity and self-loathing with relaxation. I came to know that relaxation is the bodily experience of Love. Where there is relaxation there is Love, where there is Love, there is health. Even with this insight, it would still take me many years to understand it and live it more fully, but one glimpse is all it takes sometimes to keep you on the path. I am committed to this ongoing process which has been sprinkled with many more glimpses into deep peace and self acceptance.

Let It Be Enough

Although I was getting closer to understanding how to maintain health and happiness, I was still subconsciously driven by a feeling that I had to prove something to the world and myself. It wasn't enough to show up every day and do good work, because I didn't think I was ever going to be good enough, so I kept striving. It took me a while to accept that I am not cut out for that kind of striving. In the years after moving back to New England I spread myself out in many directions until I was spread so thin I almost came apart. I created a massage curriculum for a technical school in my town, started a free massage clinic for veterans, and helped start two wellness centers. I also made my way through three more intensive bodywork and yoga trainings on both coasts, maintained a full time bodywork practice and began teaching yoga and meditation. In time I added being in the dance studio several nights a week to my roster. After years of contemplation and driving myself to exhaustion, I've come to know that showing up each day and doing your work to the best of your ability is enough. Often times your work cascades much further than you will ever know. There is contentment to be had in mindfully bringing your gifts and talents on a small scale to those around you. It is not necessary to be rock star famous to have an effect. Regardless of what our obsession with famous people has done to our feelings of self worth, everyone who realizes their passion—and then offers that passion to even one person, adds tremendous value to our society as a whole. The unity and friendship of real human contact in small town communities are the heartbeat of any civilization. What you contribute to your community each day builds a legacy. In the movie, *It's A Wonderful Life,* we see a poignant example of this. Jimmy Stewart's character wanted to go off to exotic lands and travel the world, he wanted to be a hero. He didn't want to take over the family business at The Savings and Loan and stay in his home town. Then he gets a glimpse, one fateful night, into what his home town would become without his presence. When we are shown all of the things that would have happened if Jimmy's character, George Bailey, had never existed, we understand he is indeed a hero. It may not look like what he thought it should, but he is a hero regardless. His kindness, generosity and community spirit kept Bedford Falls a thriving cooperative place with the other fate of a corporate take-over of the town ultimately thwarted by his presence. The wisdom and value of every person who becomes part of a community matters. One life can touch people in such important and meaningful ways. Quality connection with a manageable number of people is a primal necessity even if technology urges us to abandon our primal needs. We can choose to stand firmly in honoring the deep roots of our collective humanity and embrace moderation and balance in terms of technology. Exhausting yourself trying to prove to the world you are fabulous can rob you of being in the present moment. We will look in depth at the effects of social media, and the lure of 'celebrity envy' later on in this book. Maybe you will find more meaning and freedom in returning to more face to face connection with a handful of well known and trusted comrades, instead of also trying to manage hundreds of virtual acquaintances and living most of your life immersed in a virtual reality. Social media has its place, it can be a useful tool for building a business and getting information out there. However it can also become an illusory world of half truths, constant comparison of yourself against others and eventual loneliness from lack of real connection.

In Summary

Every where I've been, I see some universal themes among our fellow humans. We can tend to be hard on ourselves and deep down inside we do not think we are good enough. We judge, make up stories, and at all costs try very hard not to be wrong. We love sugar, fast food, alcohol and are addicted to electronic devices. We are plagued by constant chatter and chaos within our minds that wears us out prematurely and brings us depression and anxiety. We are living in ways that are inhospitable to continued life upon this planet both for individuals and the collective whole. Many of these trends become a factor in our health and well being. I make no claims to any absolutes, only themes that come up consistently among myself and those I have come in contact with over the course of life. It is in my nature to observe continually and so some of what I hope to offer here are the sum of those observations both as a human being and as an alternative health care practitioner. My goal for myself and for others is to restore a sense of health and sanity after the ravages of modern living has worn much of it away. This book is the expression of resolving some of the cultural belief systems that did not make sense or bring depth, health, and meaning to my life. If you find a few things within these pages that get you thinking or inspire you in small but steady ways to reclaim and restore the joy of simple living, I hope you pass the concepts on to those around you and know that your ideas and actions have an impact.

We are humans, made of glorious potential and healing power which has been buried deep under lies and irrational fears for far too long. The Calvary isn't coming to save us from ourselves. There is no magic bullet, drug, or sugar laden treat that will bring you real wellness. We are one resonating, pulsating, human family, and we need each other to be healthy more than ever now. The South Africans have a philosophy called *Ubuntu*. Ubuntu: *I am because we are, and I see you.* We are individuals and must take responsibility for our own lives, but we belong to a greater whole to which we also have a responsibility. There is a fundamental human need to be seen and cherished by our tribe even though many of us no longer live in a traditional tribal society per se. We can help each other stay true to the basic principles of humanity not only for ourselves personally, but for each other and the planet. In ubuntu societies, if you meet up with someone walking the same direction as you, it is expected that you walk together for a time until your paths naturally diverge. This way you enjoy the company of another person and are assured safety in numbers. We are part of the human family no matter what. We are walking the road together, so for yourself and for all of us, reconnect with what brings meaning into your life. Find your contentment, your wisdom, and your life purpose—not in a pill or digital device, but within your own body, heart, and mind. Through slow, consistent lifestyle adjustments may you restore and utilize this powerful strength building medicine so that the world will be full of vibrant, durable, compassionate and responsible people. Imagine creating a world full of strong healthy people who care for themselves, each other and the planet—and know that your participation is greatly needed in this project. We are all key players, we are all responsible for how our story turns out.

The Disease Cycle

"We don't need a law against McDonald's or a law against slaughterhouse abuse—we ask for too much salvation by legislation. All we need to do is empower individuals with the right philosophy and the right information to opt out en masse."

—Joel Salatin

Inflammation

In recent years there has been a lot of talk about inflammation and the harmful effects it exerts when it becomes a chronic problem. The root causes of many of our modern day afflictions is the body trying to protect itself from the onslaught of pro-inflammatory substances that have entered our food supply. We have polluted the filtration and elimination process of the body leaving many people in a chronic state of systemic inflammation. We will look at the inflammation process in more detail a little later in this chapter, but first lets us examine the role that the food industry plays here.

In part the increase in chronic inflammation has been driven by a worldwide push to produce an abundance of cheap food stuffs with the hope of feeding the ever increasing number of people living upon this planet. As time goes on, it is clear that many of the substances being added to our food supply are not tolerated well by the human body. For example, preservatives, refined sugars, flavor enhancers, and appetite stimulants have been increasingly added to many every day food items across the United States to keep them stable during travel around the world, and of course to make them tasty. Real food is tasty; it does not require flavor enhancers and appetite stimulants to be delicious, but many people no longer have a taste for real food. Instead the flavors and addictive nature of salt, sugar, and fat have become more enticing. In his bestselling book called, *Salt, Sugar, Fat: How the Food Giants Hooked Us,* Michael Moss explains at length how food scientists use the latest technology to calculate the "bliss point" of sugary beverages, making them highly addictive. He also explains how fat is chemically enhanced to make the texture feel better in the mouth which makes it harder, for example, to eat just one potato chip. The kind of fat in these processed foods is not the healthy kind of fat, but is highly processed and poorly assimilated by the human digestive tract. In a word: poison. Even the FDA is considering a ban upon these refined fats because they are known to cause disease.[2] Unfortunately, the fast pace of modern life has made cooking at home more difficult and eating these cheap, ready-to-go foods far too easy. These foods are nutritionally deficient, they are known allergens, known inflammatory agents, and are full of empty calories that are driving the obesity and diabetes epidemic. Yet, they are every where.

We are also seeing massive distribution of wheat, soy, and corn products in grocery stores, cafes, restaurants, and coffee shops. There are new varieties of breakfast, lunch, and dinner foods, all wheat, corn, and soy based, to grab and take on the run. Let us not even mention the litany of snacks readily available for the taking. These foods are the

---

2   http://www.fda.gov/ForConsumers/ConsumerUpdates/ucm372915.htm

staple of the Standard American Diet. They are quick-growing, cheap food ingredients that have a certain versatility to them. Binders, fillers, flavor enhancers, and preservatives make the process of shipping these frequently manipulated products cheaper and more convenient.

As of this moment we understand very little about the effect genetic modification has upon food, yet wheat, corn, and soy have been highly genetically modified regardless of a lack of rigorous scientific inquiry.[3] If we wait for science to blow the whistle, it will be too late. Right now agritech companies like Monsanto, Pioneer and Syngenta have protected themselves from scrutiny. Their lobbyists and lawyers have found ways to manipulate the judicial process and laws have been passed forbidding publication of independent research upon genetically altered seeds.[4] Research on genetically modified seeds is still published if the seed companies have approved of them.

Many scientists working upon these issues have expressed a serious concern after experiments, with the implicit go-ahead from the seed companies, were later blocked from publication after the results proved the seeds are not safe.[5] I see the effects this food has upon the digestion of my fellow humans and I do not like what I see at all.

Wheat, corn and soy have now been genetically modified to grow faster and resist drought, bugs, pesticides, and bacteria. The thicker hull on the wheat may resist various problems inherent in the growing process, but no one has really stopped to test what it does to the germ of the wheat or what happens when the end product reaches the human digestive tract. It will fill us up, sure, but at what expense? Can we even digest it? Dr. William Davis, a preventative cardiologist in Milwaukee, believes not. His bestselling book *Wheat Belly* is a diatribe upon the

---

3   http://www.ers.usda.gov/data-products/adoption-of-genetically-engineered-crops-in-the-us/recent-trends-in-ge-adoption.aspx#.UvUIXHnoboA
4   http://www.independentsciencenews.org/about-independent-science-news/
5   Independent Science News c/o The Bioscience Resource Project PO Box 14851-6869 Ithaca, NY 14850 USA

inflammation-causing effects of genetically modified wheat that will have you throwing away every box of pasta and muffin mix in your cupboards. One of the most pressing issues Dr. Davis points out is that the accumulation of fat around the belly is the result of consuming foods that trigger insulin, the fat storage hormone. Wheat products such as bread, pasta, muffins, crackers, and cereals are high glycemic foods which means they break down into sugar and enter the blood stream very quickly causing a spike in insulin to get that sudden flood of sugar in the blood back to a manageable amount. Unlike fat in other body areas, fat around the organs in the belly provokes inflammation, distorts insulin responses, and issues abnormal metabolic signals to the rest of the body.

As far as corn and soy, neither of these foods are meant to be consumed in high amounts yet we are eating them in huge quantities. In traditional Asian cuisine soy is more of a condiment than a food staple but the food industry here in the United States has touted the health benefits of soy, creating hundreds of products made for our consumption. Soy is also a phytoestrogen (plant estrogen) that has been linked to estrogenic breast cancer. Corn has very few nutrients and is not easily digested. Heaven only knows what soy and corn do inside the body after being genetically altered.

While world governments herald the newest technologies in mass produced food to feed the hungry, they seem to ignore the slippery slope ahead; inflammatory disease, obesity, and malnutrition are becoming epidemic. The Feeding America organization, which has partnered with big banks, food distributors, and other corporations around the world, has even placed the image of a grain of wheat right into their logo. The message is clear: mass produced grain is the Holy Grail of our salvation, the end to hunger. It is a noble cause with a hidden consequence that we all need to be aware of. Bellies may get full on the stuff, but obesity, malnutrition, and inflamed colons are little better than hunger, especially when this modified grain is now the norm not just for developing nations but worldwide. This is not your grandma's generation of grain; in fact it is hardly the same genetic seed as even twenty years ago. It grows quick and travels well, but it is almost indigestible and creates overweight yet undernourished people with highly inflamed digestive tracts. Huge agribusiness farms cannot possibly employ mindful and safe growing practices and still produce the volume of food they are expected to produce. The genetic engineering of a stronger, thicker and faster growing wheat thrills food distributors and governments which were fretting that we may not be able to feed everyone. It is all about cheap and fast, not nourishing and safe. It seems to me that convenience and food may not go hand in hand. The main reason for eating is not convenience—it is nourishment. Now, let us have a deeper look at inflammation.

Inflammation

Inflammation is the body's way of ridding itself of irritating substances such as industrial chemicals and processed foods. When a foreign and irritating element has entered the blood stream and organ tissue, the immune system will begin to heat things up in an attempt to destroy the offender. We have all seen the redness, pain, and swelling associated with physical injury. That same process also occurs in blood vessel walls and organs when an assault takes place inside of the body. The capillaries that supply blood to the damaged region dilate and increase blood flow, a necessary process that brings healing and nutrition to damaged tissues and cells, *unless* it becomes chronic in nature. In that case it is just irritating, creating the mucous that we often see in conditions like chronic sinusitis and intestinal abnormalities. All that blood dilating the capillaries creates a permeability of capillary walls so that fluid and blood proteins can move into the spaces between tissues. In short term situations this is not damaging. It becomes a problem, however, when inflammation becomes chronic causing the arterial lining to become weakened beyond repair.

As inflammation cycles begin, neutrophils and macrophages (white blood cells that eat up debris), migrate out of the capillaries and small veins and then move into interstitial spaces, which causes the familiar swelling and heat we know as inflammation. Again, this is all a necessary biological process in the short term, but inflammation is not something the body ever meant to become an ongoing state of existence. Inflammation is an immune response; it is the army of defenders inherent in all living systems designed to protect the host. Abuse it, and your immune system will in time, turn against itself, and be unable to recognize friend from foe. Autoimmune illnesses of all kinds are a result of this, every thing from allergies to thyroid disease. The body may turn on itself in other ways as well, if chronic inflammation is left uncontrolled you may find yourself with conditions like, heart disease, arthritis, gout, diabetes, chronic sinus problems, chronic headaches, hormonal disturbances, irritable bowel disease, and the list goes on right to Alzheimer's disease and even some kinds of cancer. Inflammation can happen in the gut, the brain, the lungs, nasal passages, skin and organ tissue, you name it. Your specific genetics and lifestyle habits will determine how your body will express the effects of inflammation.

Inflammation and Insulin

Eating food that produces an inflammatory response can cause a variety of degenerative diseases, among the most common of which are heart disease and diabetes. To avoid these diseases insulin levels must remain steady. If there is too much insulin spiking up and down in your blood stream, you will be more prone to inflammation and to storing that disruptive visceral fat around organs as well as developing plaque within arterial walls. Because insulin is a fat storage hormone losing weight will also become more difficult.[6,7] I am not in a war against fat,

---

6   www.health.harvard.edu/fhg/updates/Abdominal-fat-and-what-to-do-about-it.shtml
7   Craig Freudenrich, PhD: *How Fat Cells Work, How Stuff Works*, 25 July 2008

so please don't get me wrong. Abdominal fat is not in itself caused by eating fat, but by the combination of eating fat, simple carbohydrates and sugars together in the same meal over many years. Visceral fat attracts toxins, disturbs hormonal balance, and promotes inflammation. Scientists now report that visceral fat pumps out immune system chemicals called cytokines that produce tumor necrosis factor and interleukin-6, both of which play a role in cardiovascular disease and cancer.[8] These and other biochemicals are thought to have harmful effects on cells' sensitivity to insulin, blood pressure, and blood clotting.

Another reason excess visceral fat is so harmful is its close proximity to the portal vein, which carries blood from the intestinal area to the liver. Substances released by visceral fat enter the portal vein and travel to the liver, where they can alter the production of blood lipids. This is why visceral fat is also linked with higher total cholesterol and LDL (bad) cholesterol and lower HDL (good) cholesterol. There are healthy, life-giving fats offered in abundance in nutrient-rich foods, but the way the body processes fats and sugars will vary greatly depending on the food combinations your body is being given as fuel.

Triglycerides

When you eat, your body converts any calories from fats and carbohydrates that it doesn't use right away into triglycerides which are a kind of transportation fat that spreads itself all around the body. Keep in mind that the body will use the sugars and refined carbs for fuel first because they are quick burning and easier to use than fats and proteins. Over time your metabolic system will get weak and sluggish from low quality and far too-easy-to-burn fuel, if we want strong metabolism we must give the body some work to do. We want the metabolic system to work a little harder with slow burning fuel so it will stay strong. Fast burning fuel will also bog down the pancreas which will become

---

[8] *Inflammation Linked to Certain Cancers,* Journal of Clinical Investigation (JCI). June 2, 2008

exhausted from constantly producing the insulin needed to bring those sugar levels down. Over time the environment for metabolic syndrome or worse—diabetes, may set in. Refined sugars and carbohydrates are really a poor source of bodily fuel because they cannot offer sustained power. You must keep eating them to avoid the tiresome cycle of crashing blood sugar and hunger, but the more you eat them, the more inflamed, hungry and overweight you will become as you age. So start eating complex carbohydrates (vegetables), good fats, (like avocado, olives, nuts, and coconut products) and high quality protein. They are far better options to age well and avoid illness and decay. Vegetables, protein and fat sustain, and they digest slower so you feel full longer. No snacking between meals needed!

If you regularly eat more than you burn, particularly "easy" calories like refined sugars and carbohydrates combined with the low quality processed fats found in packaged fast foods, you may be heading towards high triglycerides. By now most of us understand that high triglycerides are a leading marker for heart disease. Therefore, eating a lot of high fructose corn syrup, sugar, and refined carbohydrates in combination with fats and proteins is the fast track to clogged veins and arteries which will pollute your blood and organs, and over time create widespread systemic inflammation—and not a lot of time either. The main biological job of triglyceride lipids (fats) is to store and transport energy and to give some level of structural integrity to the membranes of cells. Lipids like to combine with other stored fats and then transport that fat around via the blood vessels. However, if too much is spread around, it will lead to fatty plaque buildup in and around organs and other vessels of the body—fun isn't it? This process leads to chronic inflammation as the plaque deposits scrape against the vessel walls. If that plaque breaks off and starts to move around it may get stuck, cut off blood flow, and cause a heart attack or stroke. This scraping and inflammation within arterial cavities also creates the environment for oxidative stress on the molecular level and can actually disturb the balance of electrons within the body by creating free radicals.

Free Radicals

Well functioning molecules contain an even number of paired electrons while free radical molecules contain an uneven number of unpaired electrons.[9] These free radicals are always looking for a correction and will attack other healthy molecules in order to replace their lost electron so they can re-stabilize. By robbing an electron from a healthy molecule, the original free radical creates a new free radical. This scavenging of electrons is part of the inflammation process and will eventually result in oxidative stress and damage to healthy tissues. This promotes disease and decay and accelerates aging on the molecular level, the disease cycle starts way before symptoms show up. By the time symptoms show up, we can be sure the damage has been going on for quite some time.

This all sounds a little scary, but worry not, because we all have the power to neutralize free radicals by eating lots of fresh produce, berries, good quality protein and taking in a few extra nutrients that are antioxidant in nature, like vitamins C and E. Of course staying away from inflammatory processed foods is a key to reducing oxidation. In the chapter called "Touch the Earth" there are more tips on neutralizing the effects of free radical stress by getting onto the earth with your bare skin as a way of replacing those lost electrons. Once again the earth supports the healing and restoration of human systems. This has been true since the beginning of time.

We are now learning that inflammation is the root of many of today's most common illnesses. When your bodily intelligence detects inflammation, it tries to deal with it in the form of the symptoms commonly known as disease. Inflammation is really just your body's way of telling you to knock it off! It is a request for a lifestyle correction, not a pill. Inflammation and plaque build up disrupt proper biological processes

---

[9] Halliwell B and Gutteridge JMC (1999) Free Radicals in Biology and Medicine, 3rd edn. Oxford: Clarendon Press.

and disturb waste removal, hormone balance, and nutrition absorption. Over time these symptoms, caused by faulty lifestyle habits, create a situation where metabolic process cannot function well. This creates fatigue, bloating, weight gain, and impairs proper endocrine function so you feel sluggish, tired and old, often way before your time. Lifestyle illness, yep, that is what it is, not "heart disease" or "diabetes" but "lifestyle disease."

> *"Nothing offends patients more than to be asked to change their habits of life. Their desire is to be able to break every known law of health; then when they are called upon to pay the penalty, they expect complete absolution in a bottle or two of medicine. They are content to be patched up sufficiently to continue their practice of self-indulgence in various forms."*
>
> —Dr. Alexander Bryce

Turn It Around

I would like to encourage every reader here to reconsider the idea of convenience over quality when it comes to eating. If you have access to real food, please, eat real food. Real food is that which grows from the earth in its most natural form. If it comes in a package, read those labels. Be your own Food and Drug Administration, use your powers of assessment and common sense and choose food that nourishes over food that is simply quick, filling, and tasty. The fewer the ingredients the better, keep it simple and start preparing food at home at least a few days a week. If you must eat grain, go for older less tampered with options like millet, amaranth, and spelt. Try sprouted grains like the Ezekiel products that the "Food for Life" company offers. The lovely quinoa is also a good alternative to wheat. Personally, I do not eat grains at all with the exception of the occasional helping of quinoa which is a chenopod, harvested more for its seeds than its grain.

I find the most restorative way to eat is in the manner that does not offend our human evolutionary intelligence. This is a model which has been embraced by health enthusiasts all over the world. The terms Paleo Eating, The Primal Blueprint and The Ancestral Food Movement have been coined to name this return to deep respect for our ancient ancestry. This way of eating has captured my attention and admiration for its wise council regarding the over consumption of processed foods and refined carbohydrates in particular as well as reminding us we are of this earth and we must return to a simpler and more respectful way of being if we want to thrive in the crazed pace of modern life. You can learn more about Ancestral Health here: www.ancestralhealth.info.com

If you are looking for some inspiration (who doesn't need inspiration?) check out the wonderful documentary by Joe Cross called: *Fat, Sick and Nearly Dead. www.fatsickandnearlydead.com.* In the movie, Joe chronicles his journey from being over weight and suffering from an autoimmune disease to being completely healed, slim and much happier. He accomplishes his goals through changing his poor eating habits and sedentary lifestyle. He starts with a sixty day juice fast which effectively re-trains his taste buds to want real food all while cleaning up his blood and organ tissue and obviously allowing his weight to completely normalize. We watch Joe transform his entire life through getting off what many of us would call, "The Standard American Diet." Joe is from Australia; but few are immune now from this fast food lifestyle that has taken hold across the globe. Armed with his juicer in the back of his car, he extracts himself from his fast paced, unsustainable lifestyle and embarks upon a remaking of his life and his health. I found myself cheering for Joe and the people he meets along the way as they come face to face with their patterns of self-destruction. In the end, Joe and his friends choose health and wisdom and they begin to thrive and love life again.

Eat Local Food!

Purchasing your food from local, small family farms will help avoid the unknown factors in the factory produced mainstream food supply from wreaking havoc upon your health. Local food is fresher and more nutrient dense because it does not need to travel in a truck thousands of miles to get to you. You can visit your local farm, observe their farming practices, and see what is really going on in the growing process of your food. With giant agribusiness farms there is simply no way to know the manner in which they grow food, but chances are the focus is on cheap and fast, not nutritious and safe. Community Coop farms are also sprouting up all over the place if you want even more influence over what goes into your body. Coop Farms offer the opportunity to create your own garden but if that seems like too much work, farmers' markets are enjoying a comeback as the public becomes less trusting of the big business of growing food. See the chapter highlights for information that will help you find local farms and farmers' markets in your area.

Superhuman Healing Is Your Birthright!

Amp up your intake of dense high quality nutrition, get rid of the inflammation, and watch what happens to your ability to heal. Watch the disease cycle resolve when you interrupt it with a steady intake of pure life force from the foods that human beings were made to run on. Watch your body become a powerful healing machine. With the smallest bit of support, watch how colds disappear, skin gets smooth and glowing, and wrinkles soften. Watch your gut digest with ease and enjoy regular elimination of waste. Enjoy well working organs that are free of fatty deposits that disrupt proper functioning. Watch the excess weight fall off and see how you can be restored to the superhuman that you are. Energy will return, mental outlook will improve, and your quality of life will sky rocket. Your body was made to restore itself.

THE DISEASE CYCLE

With very little intervention most symptoms, if caught in time, will be cleared up through your body's own healing abilities. This is natural law; believe it, test it for yourself, and let me know what happens.

Chapter Highlights and Suggestions

Inflammation causes most of the lifestyle illnesses people deal with. Sugars, refined carbohydrates, and artificial, poor quality food stuffs are at the heart of the problem. Seek out local farms and eat real food. Avoid the ever increasing governmental push toward cheap crops and destructive farming practices, not to mention the folly of genetic modification of our food supply. We will talk more about this in the chapter called "Nourishment."

- Stay away, as much as you can, from refined carbohydrates and sugars.

- Ask your doctor every year for a lipid profile blood test and inflammation marker tests such as: Erythrocyte sedimentation rate, C-reactive protein, and plasma viscosity, which are blood tests tests that will detect inflammation. Watch your lipid profile test numbers if they are going up your diet will need to change.

- Check out the documentary by Joe Cross called: *Fat, Sick and Nearly Dead* for inspiration!

- Find local farms all over the country here: www.localharvest.org/

- This wonderful book will inspire and uplift you about the vital importance of local small family farms: *Gaining Ground: A Story of Farmers' Markets, Local Food, and Saving the Family Farm* by Forrest Pritchard.

- Don't blame fats for disease! Studies clearly show that good fats are essential nutrients. However, DO NOT eat them with refined carbs! The body will use the fast burning carbs and store the fats. Good fats break down slowly and keep you feeling full so you do not need to snack on crackers and chips.

- Insulin is the fat storage and inflammation hormone, so keep your glucose (sugar) levels steady so your pancreas doesn't have to work so hard to keep your sugar levels balanced. No metabolic syndrome and diabetes for you!

Ideal Glucose Levels

- Before meals—between 70 and 130 mgs
- One to two hours after meals—lower than 180 mgs
- Fasting at least eight hours—between 70 and 130 mgs

Fats

Saturated fats and trans fats create plaque and increase your risk for heart disease. However, monounsaturated fats and polyunsaturated fats are good for you, lowering cholesterol and reducing your risk of heart disease. Eat them in the absence of refined carbohydrates and watch your health return!

Good Fats

- Hemp oil
- Coconut oil
- Pasture raised butter
- Olive oil
- Fish oils/Omega 3

Not So Good Fats (trans fats)

- Hydrogenated Vegetable oils
- Soy oil

- Corn oil
- Margarine

Most snack and commercial dessert foods and baked goods contain these unsavory fats as does fast food like, McDonalds, Kentucky Fried Chicken, Burger King and Wendy's. Cook at home as often as you can.

The Placebo Effect and the Power of the Mind to Heal

"Seek the outstanding mental conflict in the person, give him the remedy that will overcome that conflict and all the hope and encouragement you can, then the virtue within him will, itself do all the rest."

—*Edward Bach*

There may come a time, in the not so distant future, that healing will take place primarily through a correction of our thoughts, actions and beliefs. We may come to understand that the human mind is among one of our most powerful human endowments, and that we can use it to create health or disease, happiness or despair. Dr. Ted Kaptchuk, who is the director of the Program in Placebo Studies and the Therapeutic Encounter at Harvard, has been studying the placebo effect, a principle that the human brain can, through belief, unleash a cascade of healing brain chemicals with an inert substance being administered to the patient. The placebo effect has been a curious occurrence that has not been fully understood or studied. Although more research is needed, the current implications are intriguing and worth our sincere consideration as they point to the tremendous power of the mind to heal a myriad of disorders ranging from pain to depression.

Kaptchuk and his colleagues found that the placebo effect greatly enhanced pain relief in migraine sufferers who had the expectation they were getting an effective drug, compared to when they took the active drug with the incorrect label "placebo."[10] Upon further investigation studies showed the release of pain relieving opioids in the brains of patients treated with placebos, which indicates that the placebo effect is a true biological phenomenon. In another study Kaptchuk set out to investigate whether placebo effects can experimentally be separated into three components: assessment and observation, a therapeutic ritual (placebo treatment), and a supportive patient-practitioner relationship.[11] The study then considered if these principles could be combined to produce incremental clinical improvement. The study was conducted with 262 adults diagnosed with irritable bowel syndrome over a six week period of time. At the three week mark assessment was made, and subjective improvements in symptoms where at sixty-one percent. At the six week mark with final outcomes being at fifty-nine percent improvement, the conclusion stated that: "Three components of the medical encounter can be progressively added to produce incremental improvement in symptoms." Another significant observation was that the therapeutic relationship between patient and physician played a role in healing:

> *"Placebo effects produce statistically and clinically significant improvement, and the patient-physician relationship is the most robust component of the placebo effect."*

---

[10] Nauert, R. (2014). How Drug & Placebo Are Given Can Enhance Migraine Relief. *Psych Central*. Retrieved on January 31, 2014, from http://psychcentral.com/news/2014/01/09/how-drug-placebo-are-given-can-enhance-migraine-relief/64275.html

[11] Components of placebo effect: randomised controlled trial in patients with irritable bowel syndrome BMJ. 2008 May 3; 336(7651): 999–1

We cannot underestimate the healing power of the human mind and the contribution of the therapeutic relationship as a fundamental component in the process of healing. There is an innate human desire to be seen, to be understood and to feel the care of a trusted guide along the path to healing. When the forces of patient participation are combined with a true desire and belief in healing, and the presence of a caring and skilled practitioner, the atmosphere and effect of healing is greatly enhanced. The current model of a visit to the primary care doctor is often just the opposite. Not only is there a feeling of being rushed, but thoughtful questions and concerns are often not taken seriously and the patient does not feel seen, heard or understood by their doctor. There is often simply not enough time to get the whole story from the patient. Couple that with very little support and follow up once the patient leaves the office, and it is no wonder the health care system is failing too many people. When it comes to the medicine of prevention and lifestyle change, a team approach and ongoing support outside the office is critical. Patient observation and input is an important part of the process. Inspiration, creativity and support need to be firmly in place. It is no wonder that alternative medicine is on the rise. Alternative practitioners are often not beholden to insurance companies in terms of how much time they can spend with people or what methods they can use. They are often highly educated, creative, compassionate and intuitive types who have been on their own healing paths and have not lost their passion and deep desire to see people get-*and stay* well. On the contrary the current mainstream medical model rewards doctors when their patients get and stay ill, driving people deeper and deeper into the system.

Heal Thyself

Several years ago I came across a lecture given by Edward Bach who was a bacteriologist from England. His lecture was given to a group of homeopathic physicians in 1931 at Southport, England and titled: *"Ye*

Suffer From Yourselves." As I read through his words, I felt the truth and beauty of his insights. His words clarified for me the nature of suffering and the potential for healing within each and every one of us. He spoke of honest self reflection, the divergence from our Divine potential and our sovereign right to freedom from oppression, both from ourselves and others. He had a high regard for personal responsibility. He believed in adherence to natural law being wiser than the laws of mankind. That no one should seek to control or oppress their fellow humans, that we should seek first to correct faulty thinking and behavior in ourselves before we look to judge another. Bach believed that what heals is love, beauty and truth. He held the belief that to bring down a virtue would neutralize a fault and offer healing. If the fundamental error in behavior is allowed to remain, inevitably the problem would occur again in an ever changing manifestation of symptoms, until the person understood how to correct their erroneous thoughts and behaviors:

> *"The treatment of tomorrow will be essentially to bring four qualities to the patient.*
>
> *First, peace: secondly, hope: thirdly, joy: and fourthly, faith."*
>
> —*Edward Bach*

The more I open my mind to expansive views about healing, the more hopeful I become and the more I feel that we are truly meant to be robust, self healing miracles of life. The human body is made to heal itself if we, with our fears, self loathing and negativity could only get out of the way. If we could: *"bring down those healing virtues of beauty, love and truth."*

Each and every one of us has a responsibility to ourselves to remember our origins. To seek those virtues and talents inherent within us and to have faith and trust that we are powerful enough to drench ourselves in that which is life affirming, gentle and restorative. Once we have reunited with this original state of health we would naturally want to be guides for our fellow humans to also find their way back to their own internal healing power—if that is what they seek. In the words of Edward Bach:

> *"To flood our natures with the particular virtue we need, and wash out from us the fault which is causing harm. Like beautiful music, or any gloriously uplifting thing which gives us inspiration, to raise our very natures, and bring us nearer to our Souls: and by that very act, to bring us peace, and relieve our sufferings."*

Bach went on to develop what he called "The Twelve Healers." They were the fundamental beginnings of what we now know as "The 38 Bach Flower Remedies."[12][13]

> *"They cure, not by attacking disease, but by flooding our bodies with the beautiful vibrations of our Higher Nature, in the presence of which disease melts as snow in the sunshine."*

Over many years of careful observation Edward Bach worked with plants, flowers and trees as his teachers. The plants themselves showed to him, as they have shown to the sensitive among us since the beginning of time, how they are designed to heal. He listened in ways perhaps more akin to a primal remembrance. That kind of listening is a sacred kind of listening that brings us into a direct communion with the laws of nature, which above all, cannot be disputed. He got still and quiet and let the answers wash over him. Then he went back to his laboratory and experimented on himself, his staff, his family, and later the community around him. He homeopathically prepared the essence of the remedies and after observing a person for some time, would administer

---

12   http://www.bachcentre.com/index.php
13   The Bach Flower Remedies by Edward Bach

a remedy and then wait. Over time the patient would come back with the next layer of suffering revealed. By this slow and thoughtful process the truth of what a person really thinks and believes would slowly be revealed. A certain level of health would return, peace would be amplified within the patient and disease would melt; *"as snow in the sunshine."* Edward Bach often observed that people are one way inside, but show a different face to the world. The secret fears we all carry can create a giant chasm of lies within our hearts and minds. This internal conflict that slowly eats away at our inner peace, eventually has the power to create physical illness. The essential disharmony between who we really are and who we show the world, can be at the root of pain, illness and suffering. Bach was after the truth, he wanted to know what was eating away at people from the inside out. He knew the power of the mind to create disease or nurture heath.

It seems to me that as we evolved as a species and as part of this earth, our cures—wrought by nature, came right along with us. How could it be other wise? Do you think CVS and Walgreens came right along with us? No, the pharmacy is a relatively new phenomenon made by limited, mechanistic ideas. Not to say modern medicine hasn't done some good. Modern medicine eradicated numerous infectious diseases that plagued civilization, like polio, and lepracy and the black plague itself which killed millions of people in medieval Europe. These medicines designed to kill and maim germs alleviated life threatening illnesses and for that we must be thankful. However as we went about living out of harmony with natural law, greater and greater bacteria and viruses have been created. Germ killing drugs allowed us to continue in our folly while lessening the consequences, but we could only do this for so long before it all began to catch up with us. A more enlightened approach might be not to stray so far from the guiding principles of life as to create such suffering for ourselves, but this is how we learn and I think we have come a long way. I do not mean to inject an either/or attitude and throw all of allopathic medicine out the window. There is much about the allopathic system that is useful and medicine is evolving more with each passing year. What I hope instead to do, is get us all thinking about a middle way. A blending of heart and mind, of rational thinking and intuitive genius. To employ all our powers of observation and consideration to come up with a more well rounded and less offensive way of understanding disease and wellness. It is time for us all to understand that *prevention* is real medicine.

If we look to nature there is healing going on all the time. If left to its own, nature will always offer a cure and heal its own. Poison ivy, for example, is often times found growing right next to jewelweed. Jewelweed, if cut open at the stem, has a bit of juice in it that will neutralize the redness, and itching of poison ivy. The same goes for the poison wood tree which is very caustic to human skin if touched. Growing close to the poison wood tree you may well find the gumbo-limbo tree which will take away the burn. The earth produced both the tree that burns and the tree that heals if you should be unlucky enough to be exposed to poison wood. The elements in the poison wood tree serve a myriad of animal life, but is a threat to human skin. Us humans can't win them all! We share this earth with many other creatures that also depend on the earth for survival but the earth would not leave us to suffer for naught! The earth itself is a wonder of restorative elements. Consider for a moment that land that has been burned will simply regenerate itself if left alone. Consider that our skin heals basically all by itself if kept clean. Hair grows back after it has been cut as does fractured bone. The body knows how to heal itself if it is durable and healthy enough to do so. That impulse to heal happens best by accumulating strength in the organs, blood and physical structure and by having a strong, positive outlook upon life.

Support in healing is some times needed and for that we turn to the earth. The cures we need were given to us by the earth. For example, the bark of the willow tree has pain reducing properties and the aloe vera plant has known anti-inflammatory, anti-bacterial, and anti-fungal properties. Tea tree oil is an antiseptic, anti-bacterial and anti-fungal.

Cinnamon, turmeric, rosemary, and birch bark all have medicinal qualities to them as well. The list goes forever on and on. Mankind did not make up the concept of healing. We are living on a planet that is a cornucopia of cures growing right under our feet. We have merely been stricken by amnesia, while the earth quietly and patiently waits for us to remember who we are, and where we came from. Yet still we destroy the forests, poison the land, pollute the air and water while creating ever more chemicals, poisons, and waste to control nature and bring the earth under our own dominion, as if we know better than She.

Edward Bach and others like him were engaged in a deep process of remembering. He was in a place of reverence and humility for the earth driven by a desire to help his fellow humans. He came to believe that much of our suffering begins in our minds, when we have lost our connection to our divine origins and when we are living in disharmony with the truth and longing of our very souls. It is up to each of us to reflect upon who we are and examine the contents of our own minds. It is up to us to consdider if our lives are a true reflection of who we really are. No one else can do this for us. The resources thoughout this book are designed to support you in asking these deeper questions and bring more depth, understanding and meaning to your life.

Chapter Highlights and Suggestions

- The human mind is among one of our most powerful endowments and we can use it to create health or disease, happiness or despair.

- We cannot underestimate the healing power of the human mind and the contribution of the therapeutic relationship as a fundamental component in the process of healing.

- The human body is made to heal itself if we, with our fears, self loathing and negativity could only get out of the way. If we could: *"bring down those healing virtues of light, love and truth."*

- Let us drench ourselves in that which is life affirming, gentle and restorative.

- Consider the 38 Bach Flower Remedies as a way of getting to know and heal yourself.

- If left to its own, nature will offer a cure. Try communing more often with the earth and your own soul.

Free Will

"I wear the chain I forged in life....I made it link by link, and yard by yard; I girded it on of my own free will, and of my own free will I wore it."

—Charles Dickens

Ah free will, the gift given to humanity in place of immortality. We fight wars in the name of defending it and we are packing weapons to ensure our freedom against a tyrannical government takeover. We have a defensive attitude about anyone who infringes upon our so-called personal freedoms all while being utterly enslaved and weakened by the consequences of them.

Freedom can be risky business especially with the availability and easy access to just about anything our little hearts might desire. Considering that millions of premature deaths in this country alone come from excess and I wonder if it might be time to think about the meaning and consequence of having this ability to give in, too often, to desire. A myriad of diseases stem from overeating, drinking too much, smoking, and taking too many drugs. The consequences of which have killed millions of people. Increasingly we are moving towards cultural acceptance of a lack of self control. In fact the excessive life is widely admired. So how are we supposed to manage our voracious appetites for endless material and carnal gratification when it can be acquired at the touch of a button, a drive around the corner, or a stroll down the street? Sugary drinks and snacks are positioned strategically at every checkout counter. We are bombarded with an endless stream of magazines and commercials that create thoughts within us of need and desire. Advertisements on television, social media sites and other internet outlets are all leading us into temptation. Self control is sneered at in favor of the influx of consumerism that affluence has brought to us. Not only do we have 24 hour access to anything we desire, but many of us have the disposable income to do quite a bit of damage to ourselves in the name of personal freedom.

I've observed that many of the happiest people I know are those that do not live in excess and have a well endowed sense of moderation and discipline in their lives. In contrast to many of the unhappiest people I know who live beyond their means. They worry endlessly about finances even while they have a brand new car, a home that they cannot afford, and too many shoes, purses, kitchen gadgets and electronics than they know what to do with. Their minds are as cluttered as their material objects and they live on a very precarious fault line of pending disaster with credit cards footing the bill while they live way beyond their means. I am not advocating rigidity or compulsive control around finances, but the contentment I witness with people who are happy with what they have is heartening. If it's not broken, don't fix it. If you don't need it, don't buy it. If you can't afford it, leave it on the shelf. If you are not hungry, stop eating. What has happened to our self control, where has our will power disappeared to and how can we get it back?

The Responsibility of Free Will

"Look at the word responsibility— 'response-ability' the ability to choose your response"

—Stephen Covey

What I am proposing is a return to a high level of self respect and personal responsibility. As our social norms recalibrate away from the dogma of organized religion and depression era rigidity we must find other more enlightened and uplifting ways than the fires of hell and damnation to moderate our behavior. Can we begin to live in ways that result in the highest good for not only ourselves but the rest of the world? Of course we can, if we set our mind to it, we most certainly can. If you are anything like me, you may need some good reasons to cut back on consumption. Hopefully your health and the health of the planet are a good start and reason enough to reconsider living in ways that offend the natural order of not only your body and mind but of our precious planet earth.

I understand there is some debate if free will even exists at all. Some proclaim that we are all just slaves of our genetics, environment, primal urges, fate or destiny. On a day to day level though, most of us understand that free will is the act of making choices about what to do in the absence of external coercion, and accepting responsibility for those actions. Increasingly we seem to be snarfing at the very idea of personal responsibility and this my friends must stop.

Self Control Equals Freedom and Accomplishment

How can we shift out of the mindset that personal responsibility and moderation is a restriction? How can we begin to see that self control can lead to freedom? After all, untethered consumption feels so good in the moment! Even if we end up broke, sick and stressed out because of it. Delayed gratification takes some time to get comfortable with. Mindfulness seems like the slow coach, but why not give it a try?

> *"The difference between successful people and very successful people is that very successful people say 'no' to almost everything."*
>
> —*Warren Buffet*

The next time you have the urge to engage in a self destructive behavior ask yourself these questions:

- Am I feeling bored?

- Am I feeling lonely, sad or angry?

- Am I procrastinating?

- Have I had enough sleep?

- Am I upset or disturbed about something?

- Am I feeling like I just want to be part of something better than what I am doing right now?

This goes for everything from stuffing processed food in your mouth and shopping for things you don't need, to compulsively using your electronic devices at the expense of your longer term goals and dreams. Instant gratification often comes at the expense of greater endeavors and keeps you from your potential. If we tend to our essential needs, and get quiet enough to notice the underlying reasons for impulsive actions, we have a better chance at making choices that actually serve what is really going on instead of acting out of unconscious habit.

"Nothing vast enters the life of mortals without a curse"

—*Sophocles*

Mindfulness

Consider the practice of mindfulness as a therapeutic technique, as the act of bringing a keener state of awareness to something and as a way of not taking things at face value or responding with a knee-jerk reaction. I have in no way mastered this technique, heavens no, but I have learned to use it just a little, enough to save me from myself on many occasions.

I liken myself to a Ferrari. Highly reactionary and sensitive, I can go from zero to sixty in a few seconds. As a teenager, tap the gas and vroom! I was off. Stress hormones would rise in an instant, I was highly reactionary, angry, and defensive. I had trained myself in this way of being as a reaction to stress and uncomfortable situations. I still have it in me, it can be conjured under the right circumstances if things build up too much, but the volume knob has been turned way down and this has improved the quality of my life and my relationships quite a bit. The act of feeling I can metaphorically slow down time and space has enabled me to wait before I react. It is all just an experiment on my part. I am just trying it on for size, I am practicing whenever I can. Some times I don't do so well, but over all my reaction to desires, impulses, and circumstances has shifted enough that much of the time I am able to have self control. Over time it has become more like my normal operating system and it is not because it just happens, it is because I practice. Although I must say I have carved much of the adversarial elements out of my life as well. This isn't always possible as life can serve us some curve balls, so it is a good idea to try the delayed reaction strategy on for size. The master element of this technique is the breath.

The Breath

It's free, we own it, and we can use it any time, any where and for any reason. The minute you put your awareness on your breath, that is all there is. Keeping your thoughts on the breath takes all your attention. The breath oxygenates the blood, calms the heart rate, slows the brain waves, and leads to the increase of the Relaxation Response. The Relaxation Response, as you may have guessed, is the opposite of The Stress Response. Feel good chemicals are released into the blood stream and in a few minutes the increase of those happy brain chemicals will allow you to go from high alert to calm and aware. In the calm/aware state decisions are more thoughtful and less reactionary. Every time you resist the temptation (what ever it may be) you build strong new responses, look at this as training. Training the central nervous system to behave slower, training your brain to release mood enhancing and relaxing dopamine and serotonin and to decrease cortisol, adrenaline and epinephrine which amplify the stress response. Your central nervous system, like your muscles, needs repeated actions to retrain it out of any habit. It takes up to about thirty to forty days for any new behavior to replace other habits, so just keep at it. Although breath does calm the central nervous system within minutes, remembering to use this technique more regularly might take some time and some practice but the results are worth the effort. With a little time you can find yourself feeling less tense, more calm, and happier. You may find yourself taking spontaneous deep inhalations automatically and this will lead to clearer thinking, decreased stress hormones, better sleep, steadier emotional states, and an over all internal sense of well being. There are breath work facilitators all over the world if you want to try an hour long excursion into oxygenation. Intensive breath work classes can strengthen your respiration and naturally make your body crave more breath, so you may find yourself spontaneously taking deeper breaths after the experience. A link to a list of breath work facilitators can be found at the end of this chapter.

Another Experiment

Play with your breath for a minute. See if you can make your breath spread out your upper rib cage, see if you can fill up your brain with air and on the exhalation allow your muscles to follow the breath down and out. Inhale, and then on the exhalation get heavy through your limbs and drop your weight as the breath leaves your body. With the next inhale, send the breath up into the back of your eyes and on the exhale relax the back of your eyes and your jaw. Sounds crazy doesn't it? It isn't, the eyes take in a lot of information through out the day and they get tight. Relax your eyes and you will relax your brain. More air in the brain equals smoother thinking. With each inhalation fill something up, with each exhalation let something go. Breathing through the nose makes it easier to feel the relief in the upper regions of your body like the face and back of the neck. Breathing through the mouth can bring greater amounts of oxygen down into the lower regions of the body like the chest, belly and pelvis.

Lets try some breathing. Find a comfortable place to sit. Have a seat on a cushion, on the couch or your bed. Sit down or lay down, what ever suits you and makes you most comfortable.

Slowly and mindfully take ten breaths and let your muscles relax on your exhalations. Go ahead, I'll wait.

Did you keep your thoughts on your breath for the whole ten breaths? Did you do all ten? Were you able to relax your muscles, your eyes and your jaw? If you find you need more guidance try going to www.calm.com or buddhify.com. You'll find guided meditations there and you can set a timer for as little as two minutes and as many as sixty minutes and you will be able to choose a soothing voice to guide you through your body and encourage you to breathe. You can download the app to your phone or try it on your lap top. Gradually work up to being able to do it on your own without your device. As you do this experiment try it in some different situations. Try it next time you reach for a cigarette, or a candy bar; stop and take ten breaths instead. Try it in rush hour traffic, try it if you have trouble sleeping, or if you feel anxious. Try it in place of any habit you'd like to live without. Remember this is just an experiment you are just observing what might happen—without pressure or punishment.

Sound

Sound can be used in so many different ways. Music is therapy. Sound can heal. In so many cultures and traditions music is used as a way to mark the time, celebrate milestones, grieve, protest, pray, and heal. Rhythm, melody and harmony unite us and keep us together as one human family. It is a language we all understand and respond to in the deepest and most basic ways. People singing together, playing the drum, the flute, fiddle, guitar, or piano—in every culture in all corners of the world, music is used to mark the passages of life and to keep us human. Music is medicine and we can all make a little music, or listen to a little music to help us on our way with what ever it is we are hoping to achieve.

In the yoga tradition, mantra is a common calming technique that sets the whole body vibrating at a sweeter level. Repeating a simple word or phrase can bring the mind to a new kind of focus. There is a science to sound vibration that dates back thousands of years, the human nervous system responds to sound vibration which is evident with the way in which music has the power to bring people of all walks of life together in harmony and unity. Music is the language of the heart, and has the power to soothe even the hardest among us. Music transcends all thinking and goes straight to our most primal instincts. So sing! Hum! Recite a mantra like "relax", "calm down" or "Let It Be". Sing it out loud or to yourself until the urge or craving passes and until you feel calm and focused again. When it comes to retraining the central nervous system and well worn habits we must get creative. Try different things that match your mood or situation. Call a friend, or go for a walk. Try at least a few times not giving in to old habits and see if you can grow your Free Will muscles to be really strong and powerful. You are the master of your own life, you have tremendous power inside of you to create the feeling that brings calm, centered, wholeness into your daily rhythms. Test this for yourself and let me know how it goes.

Chapter Highlights and Suggestions

- Consider that lack of self control creates suffering and has negative effects upon your health and well being.

- Personal responsibility brings self respect and internal ease.

- Ask yourself questions about your urges before you act on them. You may be able to tend to other needs and see that the urge for excess looses its sparkle.

- Practice mindfulness, bring more consciousness to your habitual tendencies.

- Use the breath or sound or what ever else may work for you, to calm the nervous system and slow things down before you act.

- Try calm.com or buddhify.com for breathing exercises and mindfulness training.

- Try a breath class! Find a facilitator here: www.transformationalbreathing.com.

- Practice delayed gratification whenever possible.

- Start small, do your experiment and embrace the concept of consistency over time.

- Keep your long term goals in mind over instant gratification.

Nourishment (also known as "diet")

"Let food be thy medicine and medicine be thy food"

—Hippocrates

You are what you eat, nothing that you put in your body goes unnoticed by the ever communicating intelligence of every cell you possess. Over time, the habits that settle into daily meals add up and create the physical landscape of your flesh and blood. Life affirming dietary changes can be difficult to stick with while making the unhealthy habits is so very easy and comfortable.

Generally speaking we eat for more reasons than being hungry. We eat when we are sad, we eat when we are happy and we eat when we are bored. Some times we even eat when we feel shame, guilt, and loneliness. If we unconsciously eat when in these states of mind, what we ingest often reflects those underground beliefs. It requires a good dose of self awareness and patience to shift unconscious food habits and there are good reasons that dieting often does not work. Along with unconscious eating many rebel against what is perceived as a restrictive diet because it creates a feeling of being punished, and personally I think we have all been punished quite enough thank you very much. Changing your nourishment quota does not need to feel punishing and boring. Low fat, tasteless food and no desert is no way to live. Savory dishes made with local, properly grown produce can taste delicious when you have retrained your taste buds to enjoy real food and not salt, sugar and artificial flavoring. The real food that came along with us as we evolved as a species is still the best thing to make a body thrive, there is just no getting around this. The stuff that naturally springs from the earth (and is edible, some things that grow out of the earth are poisonous) is generally assimilated into vitamins, minerals, fiber, complex carbohydrates and protein easily and generously by the body. Lots of clean fresh water and clean fresh food is what our bodies were designed to run on. The ingredients that came along later as humans tampered with the food supply have been consistently proven to cause disease and decay. I am convinced that at the top of this tinkered-with food sits sugar in all its guises and concentrations. This is not a recipe book or a diet plan manual. I am instead hoping to emphasize, in a general way, that every day you have choices about what you can eat and what you cannot eat if you want to restore yourself to health. Choices turn into patterns, patterns turn into outcomes, this is a long haul way to think. Choices are like little drops of water in a bucket, over time they add up and fill the bucket totally and even to over flowing when the water adds up enough. So over time your bucket can be filled and over flowing with vibrant health, or full to the brim with poor health and eventual disease. See the next chapter for a deeper exploration of the harmful effects of sugar. Being armed with information and truth can be a motivating factor with any lifestyle change and once you know the real deal about sugar you may be inspired to reconsider just how much of the stuff you allow into your blood stream (bucket). We've looked at the processed food industry and the basic truth about the effect packaged foods have upon the body. So that leaves us with the question: what *can* we eat?

The Good News

Now that we've gone through what not to eat, lets look at what we can eat. The answer is pretty much everything else! So eat! Eat as many vegetables as you want. Eat nuts, olives, berries, avocado, soups, salads, wild rice, coconut products of all kinds. Prepare grass fed locally raised meat in moderation, eat humanely raised poultry, game meats and eggs in moderation and not next to a refined, simple carbohydrate like french fries, onion rings or a basket of bread. Eat your meats and poultry instead with a heaping pile of butter and herb laden vegetables and greens. Eat small amounts of quinoa, and sprouted grains if you can tolerate them in your digestive track. Pull out the crock pot and make stews with loads of roots veggies, onions, garlic and ginger, herbs and spices. Let them simmer away while you are at work and come home to a nutritious hot meal ready to eat. Eat any kind of greens you can get your mitts on, they are wonderful! Mixed salad greens from our local farm with a bit of garlic infused olive oil, chicken, shredded carrots, walnuts, and some cranberries is my go-to easy salad for busy afternoons. Try kale, spinach and collard greens with leeks and garlic sautéed in butter or coconut oil with a nice piece of lean chicken breast slathered in pesto! Are you getting hungry yet? Home made cobb salad and chicken stew anyone? Celery, cucumbers and broccoli dipped in guacamole, and a side of homemade soup. Or a piece of locally raised grass fed pork or beef sautéed in onions and garlic with loads of rosemary and a big pile of stir fried greens with ginger mustard dressing. Stuffed peppers, stuffed squash, or giant stuffed heirloom tomato with a big green salad. Why not some home made banana pudding with dark chocolate and whipped cream for desert? There are so many combinations that will leave you satiated, nourished and content that don't include pasta, bread, muffins, cakes, soda, french fries, pizza or anything of the kind. Eat the left overs from dinner for breakfast for a fast, nutritious start to your day. Vegetables dipped in savory bowls of hummus, guacamole, or salsa, can be a great snack. Hard boiled eggs with a little salt, pepper and mustard is good on the run if you cannot sit and eat a meal. Nuts and an apple or clementine are a tidy snack that is easy to take and run if you must, and we all must have a quick option some times. Another good on-the-run snack might be raw goat cheese or raw cheddar cheese and an apple or pear with some nuts to take the edge off between meals. I like to make large amounts of veggie soups and stews on Sundays. Throughout the week I can pour some soup into a container and bring it with me in case I get stuck and can't get home for lunch. I can drink the soup right out of the container, it's super easy and fills my body with real fuel to sustain me if the day is too busy to make lunch. Sitting down for a full meal three times a day can be a challenge so have some quick and easy food to pop in your mouth around the house and office. Thermal bags are a nice invention for bringing food to work if you don't have a fridge at your workplace. Make your own fast food. With just a little planning and forethought you can take control of what is going into your body very easily without spending hours in the kitchen. Prepare extra food every time you cook and save the left overs, get a crock pot, it is like having a cook in your kitchen while you are away. Prepare foods that are not too messy to take on the go, like sliced veggies, cheese, chicken breast, hard boiled eggs, nuts, and fruit.

Just like grandma always said, do not skip breakfast. It is the most important meal of the day. Eating breakfast jump starts your metabolism, feeds your brain, steadies your blood sugar and provides fuel to get you through until lunch so you don't go reaching for some kind of snack food from the vending machine or coffee shop. Eat a lunch that will set you up for a light dinner so you aren't eating after six o'clock in the evening. The body wants to wind down after six or seven o'clock in the evening, digestion should mostly take place in the early part of the day, while you are moving about. Eating a meal an hour or two before bed is laying the foundation for digestive problems, weight gain, lymphatic sluggishness and blood sugar imbalance. If your body isn't busy trying to digest while you sleep, it will allow for other restoration and healing to happen during the night. Sleep is a time for repair and rest, not a time for digesting. The reason we call the first meal of the day "break"-"fast" is because we are essentially fasting for about ten to twelve hours each evening, the morning is the time to break the fast. The health benefits of allowing the body a break from digestion has been established. Mice that fasted for even six hours a day stayed lean and healthy even when fed a high-calorie diet; their mouse counterparts that had access to food day and night became obese and showed blood sugar and liver problems despite eating the same number of calories.[14] So give your body a break, let your organs rest at night by not eating a late meal before bed.

How and Where Food Is Grown Matters

The source of food is becoming more important as large scale farming has increased. How produce is grown has an impact on the nutrition content. Soil is life, the microbes, minerals, and organic matter (like moss, lichen, grasses and leaves) combine and create the nutrient dense soil that produces the nutrient dense food we all need to thrive. Poorly cultivated soil makes for weak, diseased plants that need to be managed with chemicals instead of the strength the earth provides when She is in balance with the forces of the universe. Not to mention that food grown in rich, balanced, robust soil tastes so much better. Start with quality ingredients and your food will taste delicious.

Resources

The Ancestral Health Movement has cook books with savory, nutrient dense meals that take a short time to prepare. Get online and

---

14 Mark Mattson, head of the National Institute on Aging's neuroscience laboratory April 28, 2003

search these key words for cookbooks: Mediterranean Diet, traditional eating, whole foods cooking, Primal Blueprint and the Paleo diet. You will find a host of wonderful resources. Above all find the kind of real food that does not offend your digestion. When metabolism has become lazy and sluggish from eating too many quick burning processed carbohydrates over many years it can often create food sensitivities. If you have belly bloat, intestinal gas or get stuffed up in your sinuses after eating it could very well be due to poor digestion, or a food sensitivity. The lining of your colon may be inflamed and hyper permeable which means your colon needs a rest from trying to deal with processed, chemically toxic food and drink. Often times feeding your body with basic, real food in the absence of junk food will heal your organs. Some times though extra support and help is needed. You may need to increase the beneficial bacteria in your gut to help it repair and work normally again. There could be a more complex problem like gluten intolerance or more serious inflammation in the colon. If a month or so on a clean, whole food, grain free diet does not lessen your bloat, gas, or indigestion, consider seeking the guidance of a Functional Medicine doctor. At your visit tell that doctor everything that concerns you, it will help them to get the full picture of your situation. In a Functional Medicine consult you should have an hour with your doctor the first visit. They should get as much information from you as possible so they can find the best plan of action. We are all different; our chemistry, life experience, family history, and genetic coding are unique. There is no way to offer real advice without a face to face interaction, selected diagnostic tests and a little trial and error experimentation. Functional Medicine is the medicine of the future, you will find the experience quite different from the doctor of the near past. Many Functional Medicine practices take a variety of health insurance and are affiliated with labs and hospitals. You can find more information here: www.functionalmedicine.org/about/whatisfm/ You can find a list of doctors with this additional Functional Medicine training here: www.functionalmedicine.org/practitioner_search.aspx?id=117

Special Diets

People who are vegetarian may have a harder time with carbohydrate restriction. Sprouted grains and legumes can be tolerated by some people and the combination of the two can offer complete protein. If you are a vegetarian or vegan who has very bad sugar and carbohydrate cravings, and you are having bloating, gas, weight gain, or digestion problems you may want to consider that what you are eating could be the cause of it. The spiritual, ethical, environmental and political drive behind eating an all plant based diet is important and honorable and if done wisely can offer nutrition and health benefits. However I have seen many a vegetarian living on takeout Mexican food and french fries become very unhealthy in the name of being vegetarian. I have seen a gorging upon soy products, fake cheese and textured vegetable protein products that are no better in terms of health than living on pizza and McDonalds salads. The sodium count is high, the nutritional quality is low and although animals are not being sacrificed, neither are those people doing much to preserve their own lives. I've seen too many vegetarians with raging symptoms of gluten intolerance and sugar imbalance sacrificing their own health in the name of saving animals. Eagerly touting the evils of animal products while busy gaining weight and becoming pre-diabetic. I was a vegetarian for many years and I regularly consumed a plate of pasta with tofu and veggies for lunch and dinner. I ate whole wheat toast, bagels or english muffins every morning for breakfast with peanut butter and fruit thinking I was being so healthy. My blood sugar was out of control, I wasn't sleeping, and I had daily binges on sweets. No matter how much will power I applied I could not stop eating those cookies! Oh how I love cookies! Migraines were a monthly occurrence as was pain in my joints. I lived on grain of all kinds; wheat, couscous, pasta, and tortilla chips with beans or lentils. I ate piles of vegetables with starchy carbs, tofu and soy sauce. I thought I was doing the right thing, and could not understand why I felt so awful. Eventually I began to use a nutrient count program and put everything I ate into it at the end of the day. When I stopped to honestly examine the amount of carbohydrates I was consuming, it was up around three to four hundred grams per day. All burning and churning away into sugar that left me utterly fatigued, bloated, moody and plagued with migraines. Eating sugar begets eating more sugar, it doesn't matter too much what kind of sugar it is, carbs burn quick, their end result is sugar and you must get more every few hours or risk the hunger and anxiety of the blood sugar crash after the onslaught of insulin is done clearing all that sugar out of your blood. I wasn't eating a lot of processed foods, I was cooking at home much of the time except for those cookies from Whole Foods. I thought they were fine to eat because they were made with whole grains, cane sugar and organic chocolate chips. In the years that I was vegetarian I gained fifteen pounds, and became totally addicted to carbohydrates. Even though I was working out hard at the gym four days a week, doing yoga several days a week and running about three miles per day. Upon removing grain from my diet my sugar cravings began to diminish within about a week. I lost most of the weight I had gained in about three weeks. I now work out about half the amount that I was and my weight does not fluctuate like it once did. I sleep longer and deeper and my cravings are manageable. I think I've had two migraines in the past three years which is the biggest relief of all. The problem was of course, without that tofu, grain and legume combination where would I get my protein from? A girl cannot live on tofu and nuts alone! The hard cold facts hit me. I would have to find another source of protein. I am very concerned about animal welfare and the environment and it was not an easy decision to go back to eating animal products. I did some research into local non factory farmed sources for the small amount of meat, poultry and eggs I started to eat. Factory farm products have not been a part of my life for decades and I was not about to start giving a single dime to factory farms. I found two local farms who raise chickens, pigs and cattle and went over for a visit. My reverence and love for the animals that die so that I may live in vigor and good health is not ever, for one-second, lost on me. My diet is about seventy-five percent plant based with the remainder being high quality animal protein among other things like nuts, eggs and raw cheeses, berries, and homemade veggie juices from the juicer. I now enjoy real non pasteurized raw cheese around one or two times per week as a treat with no problem, but if I eat more—the sinus congestion appears. I had to play with serving size and frequency and found that once every three days or so I can have a bit of cheese and have no symptoms at all. I have found the food combinations that do not elicit any bloating, sinus congestion, weight gain or spikes in blood glucose levels. I used a glucose monitor at first until my blood sugar became stable. No doctor was ever going to tell me what I learned on my own from common sense, honest inquiry and deep listening to my body.

Diabetes runs wild in my family history so in my case the huge reduction in carbohydrates was critical. Not everyone has such reaction to high carbohydrate living but I knew I had to turn those diabetes genes off before it was too late. I pray that the animals might agree with me. In my case my biology eventually trumped my ethics and I get more and more accepting of this as time goes on. There is no sense in having any feelings of guilt as you eat, so the experience of listening to my body was a fine lesson in accepting what is.

Studies now show that refined sugars (high glycemic foods) are addictive.[15] Wheat is very high on the glycemic index believe it or not. A study published in *The American Journal of Clinical Nutrition,* reported how intake of high glycemic food is regulated by dopamine-containing pleasure centers of the brain. Much the same way any other addictive substances stimulate the "opiate" receptors of the brain, creating pleasure and a desire for more and more of the substance. In the study conducted with Dr. David Ludwig, and the New Balance Obesity

---

15   Effects of dietary glycemic index on brain regions related to reward and craving in men David C Alsop, Laura M Holsen, Emily Stern, Rafael Rojas, Cara B Ebbeling, Jill M Goldstein, and David S Ludwig from the New Balance Foundation Obesity Prevention Center, Boston Children's Hospital, Boston, MA (BSL, CBE, and DSL); Ulm University, Ulm, Germany (BSL); the Beth Israel Deaconess Medical Center, Boston, MA (DCA and RR); Brigham and Women's Hospital, Boston, MA (LMH, ES, and JMG), and Harvard Medical School, Boston, MA (BSL, DCA, LMH, ES, RR, CBE, JMG, and DSL).

NOURISHMENT (ALSO KNOWN AS "DIET")

Prevention Center at Boston Children's Hospital, the subjects consumed a high-glycemic milkshake after which a surge in blood sugar levels was noted, followed by a sharp crash four hours later. This decrease in blood glucose was associated with excessive hunger and intense activation of the nucleus accumbens, a critical brain region involved in addictive behaviors. The study concluded that a high-glycemic index meal sharply decreased plasma glucose, increased hunger, and selectively stimulated brain regions associated with reward and craving. Don't you love science? We can see so much now and funding for studies of this kind is increasing. Let us take this information to heart and make wiser choices in the spirit of self respect and love of life!

Fish

Fish is suspect sadly enough due to mankind's abominable polluting of our water. Between countless oil spills, pesticide run off, and atmospheric pollution we've done a bang-up job of creating mutated sea life, sick coral reefs and toxic waterways beyond our wildest imaginings here at home. Much of our fish comes from the Gulf of Mexico and the gulf is very sick right now.[16][17] Other countries are certainly not exempt either. Until we know more of the truth about the Fukashima Nuclear disaster I would stay away from eating any sea life coming from the Pacific. Russia and China have dumped a fair amount of toxic chemicals into the ocean as have England and Ireland. Decreasing oxygen levels in the ocean caused by climate change and nitrogen run-off, combined with other chemical pollution and rampant overfishing impedes the ability of the oceans, bays and rivers to withstand these assaults. According to the 2013 statement by The International Programme on The State of the Ocean, the earth's 'buffer' is seriously compromised

---

16 The Deepwater Horizon Oil Spill and the Gulf of Mexico Fishing Industry Harold F. Upton Analyst in Natural Resources Policy February 17, 2011 https://www.fas.org/sgp/crs/misc/R41640.pdf
17 http://www.nrdc.org/oceans/default.asp

and the oceans are deteriorating much faster than previously believed.[18] Farmed fish are no better for eating. Fish raised in farms are not fed the things that fish eat. Instead they are fed soy and corn, can you think of anything more ridiculous? Fish do not eat soybeans or corn so just what kind of fish are being raised in these conditions? Not the kind we should be eating that is for sure. Many of us think that by eating fish we are getting those heart and brain healthy omega 3's. If those farmed raised fish are eating soy and corn I can promise you they do not have a natural source of omega's in their bodies. Perhaps omega's are being added through some kind of replacement fish meal but there is so much wrong with that equation I cannot even begin to address it. These fish are being raised in an unnatural environment that is not balanced by the forces of the natural world, they are being fed junk, then they are being killed and eaten. The whole cycle is nefarious and I'd rather not see any of us supporting this method of raising fish. It is no better than the conditions our animal friends are subjected to in large factory farms.

The need for quality long chain and medium chain fatty acids for health has been established for quite some time now.[19] We need fatty acids for numerous body functions, such as controlling blood clotting and heart health, building cell membranes in the brain, and for keeping inflammation in check . Since our bodies cannot make omega-3 fats, we must get them through food. If fish is too contaminated to eat in the near future supplementation of fatty acids may become more necessary.

There are different kinds of essential fatty acids. ALA (alpha-linolenic acid) which come from vegetable sources. (another good reason to amp up your intake of green things!) The others are (EPA) eicosapentaenoic acid and (DHA) docosahexaenoic acid which come from marine sources. As our population grows and the oceans become ever more

---

18   www.stateoftheocean.org/research.cfm
19   http://nccam.nih.gov/health/omega3/introduction.htm

polluted there is concern over where those beneficial fatty acids will come from in the future. There seems to be some hopeful indications that algae provides a good source of DHA. When scientists began to study the useful properties of algae for long-term space flight they discovered a natural strain of algae that produced high levels of DHA omega-3. Harvested domestically, the algae can be grown in large stainless steel fermentors at an FDA-inspected facility. This algae is free of ocean-borne and environmental contaminants and looks hopeful as an alternative source that would not require further degradation of the ocean and sea life. See the chapter highlights below for sustainable sources of algae.

I am not telling you what to eat, I am more begging you about what *not* to eat, and it is mainly food of the refined, non nutritious, harmful variety that no one should be eating, everything else is fair game. Keep an eye on your blood sugars and energy levels. If you suffer from fatigue, dizziness, headaches, mood swings, and frequent hunger and thirst, you may have a sugar imbalance. Use a glucose monitor and work with your doctor. Above all, be honest with yourself and stay away from refined foods that degrade your health. Experiment with removing foods that you suspect may be causing reactions. Things like wine, poor quality dairy products, chocolate, wheat, corn and soy are common triggers as are some nuts, eggs and shell fish. Some times eating a food once a week can be tolerated even if it is a food you are sensitive to. Remove it from your diet for at least a full week and really watch what happens when you reintroduce it back into your diet. If symptoms return you have your answer. Try taking two weeks off and reintroduce the food again. Experiment, go ahead it is your body and you can do a lot to work with the information your body is constantly offering you. The Human Restoration Project begins with food, we cannot restore while eating processed, dead food-like substances.

Chapter Highlights and Suggestions

- You are what you eat (and drink)—so eat real food, ditch the processed stuff.

- Find fast, easy and nutritious whole food recipes that will allow you to choose highly customized options here: www.whfoods.com/recipestoc.php

- If digestive ailments do not lessen within a month of whole food eating consult a Functional Medicine doctor: www.functionalmedicine.org

- Read up on the cutting edge shift in medicine: *Functional Medicine: The Origin and Treatment of Chronic Diseases / Edition 2 by Helmut W. Schimmel*

- Try not to offend your genes, you can make them play nice with you if you adjust your lifestyle.

- Consider where your food is coming from, quality food is essential for nutrient content and safety.

- Look for alternative sources for your beneficial DHA from algae instead of fish and eat your greens and walnuts for daily requirements of ALA. Try this link for algae products from Cellana: cellana.com/products/renew-omega-3/

The Truth About Sugar

"Some of the largest companies are now using brain scans to study how we react neurologically to certain foods, especially to sugar. They've discovered that the brain lights up for sugar the same way it does for cocaine."

—*Michael Moss*

Even while indulging in sugary, artificial foods bereft of nourishment is the real punishment, it can feel so good in the moment. In my case, sugar feels like love, it feels like nurturing and it turns on things in my brain that make sugar a highly addictive substance for me. Not everyone responds to sugar in this way but for me it is like a narcotic. Maybe for you it is other forms of sugar like refined carbohydrates dowsed in salt, or sweet creamy things, or maybe it is alcohol. Bread, pasta, cereal, and a host of other simple carbohydrate based food items turn into sugar quickly and the pancreas sees little difference between a plate of pasta and a handful of cookies. Eating a diet heavy in simple carbohydrates and sugars, over a long period of time, is not the way to create ideal body composition as you age. When foods burn down into sugar quickly the body must regulate how much of it is flowing through the blood at any given time. In order to do this, insulin gets released, the fat storage hormone extraordinaire, and you are on a blood sugar roller coaster until you get the next hit of quick burning fuel. Some insulin in the blood of course, is normal and healthy, but too much, over too long, becomes destructive. Inflammation, weight gain, bloat, poor digestion and disease will be your inheritance if you are not careful. I had to admit to myself that despite the cultural acceptance of sweetness as being fun and friendly, I cannot touch the stuff on a regular basis.

As time goes on there are brave people challenging the sugar lobby and the truth about sugar is finally starting to come out despite a billion dollar, award winning marketing campaign that for decades has protected the sugar empires of the world. In an article in Mother Jones magazine's Nov/Dec 2012 issue called: *"Big Sugar's Sweet Little Lies"* we are informed about a series of events that culminates with a pair of executives from the Sugar Association stepping up to accept the Oscar of the public relations world. The award, called the Silver Anvil award, is given for excellence in the forging of public opinion. For over a decade, the sugar industry attempted to spin the mounting facts that sugar is a likely cause of obesity, diabetes, and heart disease. Industry ads convinced the public that sugar was a harmless benign substance that brought joy to all. They even went so far as to advertise that eating sugar helped you lose weight which was then brought into question by the Federal Trade Commission, and the Food and Drug Administration. Investigations were launched to inquire if sugar was even safe to eat at all. The findings of course were buried deep, the right people were paid off, and funding for real non-biased studies was halted. Many years would go by before the safety of eating sugar was ever brought into question again. For the consumer, the misinformation of this campaign to maintain the innocence of sugar means that since the end of any real inquiry into its safety in the late '70s and '80s, diabetes has nearly tripled and the number of Americans diagnosed with obesity has risen from fifteen percent in 1980 to over thirty-five percent as of 2010. In terms of legislation, like tobacco and fire arms, the lobby protecting the sugar industry takes time, money and dedication to infiltrate and as of this moment, there is very little indication that the truth about sugar will hit the main stream any time soon. Once again it is up to us to follow our gut on this one. We cannot wait for the Food and Drug Administration to do the research before we pay attention to our own evidence and experience. There are places to look for the truth, regardless of who endorses it or not.

In recent years the scientific tide has begun to turn against sugar. Despite the industry's best efforts, researchers and some brave public health authorities have come to accept that the primary risk factor for both heart disease and type 2 diabetes is a condition called metabolic syndrome. According to the Centers for Disease Control and Prevention metabolic syndrome affects more than seventy-five million people in the United States alone. In my estimation I'd say the better portion of people I see in my wellness practice, who are over forty-five years old, either have or are on their way to metabolic syndrome. The symptoms of this disorder are very frustrating and difficult to deal with. They include weight gain; especially around the abdomen, despite a low calorie diet and light to moderate exercise. They also include increased insulin levels, elevated triglycerides and a serious increase in pro-inflammatory activity through out major organs, blood and soft tissue systems. It is hard for the healing ability of the body to be activated under these conditions. The inflammation of metabolic syndrome has also been linked to various cancers and Alzheimer's disease.[20] Scientists have now established quite clearly that sugar causes metabolic syndrome and a host of other degenerative diseases. Remember our credo? If it supports life, do it, if it encourages decay and disease, stay away. Often times the metabolic syndrome that shows up in our forties is a result of a life time of refined sugar and carbohydrate consumption, but you can turn it around. So stay away from refined sugars and artificial sweeteners, and instead use small amounts of unrefined sugar in combination with

---

20 Cancer as a metabolic disease. Metab (Lond). 2010 Jan 27;7:7. doi: 10.1186/1743-7075-7-7., Shelton LM.

a plant based diet with moderate amounts of high quality proteins and most definitely treat high fructose corn syrup as the poison that it is.

High Fructose Corn Syrup

Most of the sugar we ate up until the mid 1970's came from sucrose refined from sugar beets and sugar cane. It was then discovered that distilling corn in the form of fructose, dextrose and high fructose corn syrup (HFCS) was less expensive to produce. The use of it exploded onto the scene infiltrating everything from baked goods, canned goods, juices, candy, soda and beyond. The problem with high fructose corn syrup is that it can only be metabolized in the liver and the liver quite frankly is not so thrilled with this idea. A study published by *The American Journal of Clinical Nutrition,* November 2002 found that when fed large amounts of refined fructose, laboratory animals developed fatty deposits and cirrhosis, similar to the conditions that develop in the livers of alcoholics. The unsavory effects of refined fructose varies depending on age, baseline glucose levels, and family history of diabetes, and triglyceride concentrations. So those folks with high blood pressure, insulin resistance, and high triglycerides all must become the HFCS police. Also, non-insulin dependent diabetics, people with functional bowel disease, and postmenopausal women must be on the watch and remove it from their diets.

In reality how ever, it seems clear to me that all of us might be wise to avoid exposure to refined fructose, but especially those people listed above. This does not mean don't eat real fruit. Real fruit has fiber that will slow down the sugar hit to your blood and there are vitamins and minerals to be had in fresh fruit. However, commercial fruit juices and any products containing high fructose corn syrup are more dangerous than sugar and should be removed from the diet.

Consuming high fructose corn syrup will diminish the ability of the liver, one of our most precious elimination organs, to do its job which makes it harder to loose weight and have healthy organs, blood, skin and hair. Got bloat? Liver stagnancy might be a good place to consider a cleanup project. This will relieve the strain of eliminating the toxic effects of liver congestion and encourage your lymph system to work better thereby reducing bloat and preventing disease.

So How Much Can We Have?

The Mayo Clinic suggests ingesting no more than one hundred of your daily intake of calories from sugar which is about six teaspoons per day. There are others who say it should be even less, like the Weston A. Price Foundation, who I have come to admire and trust as a forerunner of wisdom and truth when it comes to food. The Weston A. Price Foundation suggests no more than two teaspoons of sugar in the blood at all times. The Ancestral Food Movement also says we should keep our sugar intake to about two teaspoons in the blood at all times, spread out over the day; however this recommendation does not include a single drop of the refined varieties of sugar. There are natural sugars every where so not getting enough is generally not a problem. This is not to say you need to be rigid. Enjoy the sweetness in moderation and make it of a high quality non-refined nature. There are actually quite a lot of choices out there for your sweet fix. Cacao, dark chocolate, fruit, and a bit of honey or maple syrup are all of a less refined kind of sugar that if eaten sparingly within a well balanced diet can be well tolerated by most of us. If you have any inclination to do a bit of baking there are some great dessert recipes out there from the Ancestral Food Movement that are naturally sweetened, non refined, delicious desserts. Just don't eat them every day. Make dessert time something special that you do occasionally. What adds up in the wrong direction is the can of soda with every meal, the processed breakfast cereals, candy bars, cakes, cookies, bagels, and muffins that are loaded with artificial sweeteners that we need to reconsider if we want to get the metabolic fires burning again.

Chapter Highlights and Suggestions

Eating a diet heavy in simple carbohydrates and sugars, over a long period of time, is not the way to create ideal body composition as you age.

- We cannot wait for the Food and Drug Administration to do the research before we pay attention to our own evidence and experience in regard to ingesting too much sugary food and drink. Listen to your body, feed it food that will not offend your metabolic system.

- In recent years the scientific tide has begun to turn against sugar. Researchers and some brave public health authorities have come to accept that the primary risk factor for both heart disease and type 2 diabetes is a condition called metabolic syndrome caused by eating too much sugars and refined carbohydrates.

- HFCS has been shown to damage proper liver function. Read food labels you may be surprised at how many common packaged foods are full of HFCS.

- The Weston A. Price Foundation suggests no more than two teaspoons of sugar in the blood throughout the day. This does not include a drop of the refined varieties of sugar.

- Enjoy sweetness in moderation and make it of a high quality non-refined nature.

Movement and Posture

To regain our freedom let us shake off the burden of inertia.

—M. Tomaski

As a massage therapist, Structural Integration practitioner, yoga teacher and former dancer it might not come as a surprise that I consider regular movement and strong, balanced, upright posture to be medicine. The health and balance of the physical body is an important foundation for the way we express ourselves in the world and how effective we are in our daily lives. The mind, the organs, the breath, the blood, lymph and bones all function more effectively if the spine, (front, back and sides) has some strength, endurance and flexibility. The most efficient and comfortable stance is one of an upright position which allows for space and flow of physiological process instead of the slumped over spine I see so often out there in the world. Pain, stiffness and heaviness in the physical form requires a lot of energy to endure, energy we could be using for a variety of other higher functions in life.

In terms of The Human Restoration Project philosophy, movement is right up there with real food, enough rest, and connection to the natural world. Skeletal and muscular resilience and integrity can make life a buoyant joy while the lack thereof is a physical burden that follows you through your days and nights robbing you of the vital energy that could be better spent elsewhere. You deserve more, you deserve to enjoy your body, to be at ease in your place upon this earth and to allow the forces of gravity to support and enhance your experience of living in a human body. After all, the human body is a splendid work of art when allowed to express its potential. It was designed for grace, agility, and endurance. A conditioned body is a thing of great beauty as countless sculptures, paintings and poetry will attest. In all its forms the body is a glory to behold, from tall and lean, to thick, powerful and strong, to full and voluptuous. We can have vibrant health in all bodily constitutions. To commune with our physical potential is one of life's most precious gifts to us. The body wants to serve at ever higher levels and allow you to have the fullest expression of life that you can have while you are here.

Our Glorious Physical Form

Muscle tissue is incredible. It is utterly adaptable and forgiving and takes to activity at any age and in just about any condition. Our muscles are composed of water, lipids (fat), and proteins like collagen, actin, myosin, enzymes and essential and nonessential fatty acids. Depending on lifestyle choices muscle composition is variable. More fat in the muscle fibers means less water and more potential for stiffness, stagnation and toxic build-up. Insufficient protein intake can leave the muscles depleted and prone to injury. Too much sugar in the diet and the muscle will become inefficient in converting glucose to useable power and fatigue will set in. Muscle and collagen composition change not only from how the internal environment is maintained via lifestyle, but from aging and injuries as well. Genetics also influences how inherently long, short or dense our muscle fibers, ligaments and tendons are. Don't be fooled though because we most certainly have some influence over maintaining the health of these tissues regardless of genetic propensity or injuries. If hydration, suppleness, strength and nutritional health are maintained in the physical structure, life is supported by life. Moving through your days will be easier, the process of aging can be slowed down and greatly mediated. This is good news!

Fascia

All around the muscle layers of the body is a strong, white, gossamer tissue called fascia. Great stuff fascia, some have called it, *The Organ of Posture,* and no one honors that statement more than the Structural Integration community to which I belong. If you want some manual help to get more upright through your spine and maintain fluidity in your joints stay tuned for information about Structural Integration later on in this chapter.

Fascia organizes muscle fibers and strengthens and protects all soft tissues of the body. From muscles like the trapezius and quadriceps to organ tissues like the small intestines and liver, fascia is a critical structure to consider in terms of bodily function. Our entire soft tissue matrix is strongly influenced by fascia and as much as it can serve you if it is well organized and hydrated it can also bind you into faulty movement patterns, pain and stiffness if you have long habits of a sedentary nature and postural strain. Research has also shown that fascia is a communicative system that sends and receives information regarding the health of the entire body into the central nervous system.[21] Suggesting an explanation for why a weak, slumped over body correlates with depression, lack of energy and poor digestion, or why inflexibility and lack of fluidity in the physical form can translate to a rigidity of thought in the personality. Observe this for yourself while you're out there running errands or make note of posture in the people that you know. See if you notice how their posture reflects the way they think, and view

---

21 The continuum of fascia throughout the body allows it to serve as a body-wide mechano-sensitive signaling system. (Langevin, 2006)

the world. Does their world view and mental outlook coincide with the way they sit, stand and walk? A fluid, flexible, upright spine very often accompanies a person with a can-do attitude and strong internal disposition. Not every single time, as us humans are complex, but I observe this more often than not. At least outwardly those who have structural integrity tend to display an adaptable and positive out look on life.

Stiffness

Every night as you lay sleeping, at rest and dreaming away, the space between your muscles grows a layer of fine filaments of connective tissue. When you wake up, put your feet on the floor and begin to walk it may take some time before the evening stiffness wears off from this extra stuff that has been deposited while you were sleeping. As you move, that night time build up warms and becomes a bit more pliable as blood pressure increases and pumps blood through the body with a little more force. This layer of night time tissue can totally melt with targeted stretching and movement and if really thick tissue results from injury or many years of not moving enough, hands-on therapy can restore pliability to the stiff or injured parts by manually stretching, spreading and smoothing away these extra layers of binding. Unless you move in some significant way every day, this stiffness will continue to build and build until there is a palpable change in the consistency of your muscles and joints. If a lack of regard for the physical form occurs, over time healthy tissue is replaced by hard, unyielding tissue that has a thicker and denser fiber woven within it. This thicker fiber pins down your joints and makes range of motion more difficult and painful. So the quality of our aging in terms of stiffness, is the sum of movement or lack of movement plus time. How you spend that movement potential determines the quality of movement as you age. I do not believe that a general stiffness needs to accompany aging, nor do I believe that this kind of stiffness is normal. It can be a sign of neglect of the physical form but aging does not have to go that way. As years pass you may feel more stiff upon waking than you used to, or more stiff when rising after sitting for any length of time. We correlate this stiffness with aging as the deeds of our lives accumulate. Not enough movement, coupled with more acid build up from poor food choices and scarring from injuries makes stiffness more prevalent . If you eat too much sugar and acid producing processed foods stiffness is exaggerated even more, but I do not believe for a second that we should just accept this when we have been so well endowed with muscles that are designed to restore and rehydrate with even just a little bit of mindful movement, proper care and nutrition. More good news! We are living in bodies that are *The Masters of Restoration!*

You Are More Powerful Than You Think!

Changing body composition occurs fairly quickly with a bit of determination and consistency, even if you spent twenty years sitting at a desk, driving in the car a lot and sitting on the couch while munching away on packaged and processed foods. The body is delightfully accommodating. It is just our minds that have been wrongfully convinced that it is too hard and not worth it to change our habits, opting for a pill or surgery over facing our own disease enhancing habits. There are so many different kinds of movement options now, there is quite literally something for everyone thanks to human ingenuity hybridizing everything from yoga and Pilates (known as Yoga-Lates) to blending cabaret and latin style dancing, to doing tai chi on a stand up paddle board. You may try something and feel it is not for you, this is no problem because if you keep exploring, you will find the kind of movement that will suit you. If done with some commitment, movement will yield results quickly in comparison to how long perhaps you've been taking the elevator and the easy chair route. It is a good idea to find a few different ways to get moving to keep things interesting and find ways to make it enjoyable and stress reducing at the same time. Get outside whenever possible, in all seasons, because as my friend Larry says, *"there is no bad weather, only inappropriate clothing."* The more we develop aversion to the weather and being in the elements, the weaker we become. Do not fear moderate cold and heat! Dress for these events, be sure to stay hydrated, but get out there and your body, mind and spirit will get stronger! No matter what condition you are in, you can get stronger than you currently are. Again, use common sense. If you are not steady on your feet don't go strolling about on an icy sidewalk. But on a clear, but cold sunny day, get your thermals out, pull on the wool socks and go outside. Your body will adapt and become stronger if you allow it to return to the earth. Do it wisely of course. Dress well, get enough sleep, and a good breakfast and then go outside and feel the elements exert their strengthening influence upon your flesh and blood. Some times just a little more strength and ease in your body can change your entire perspective on life.

Resources

If you have injuries, are excessively stiff or afraid to move please seek professional guidance and start slowly. Physical therapists, athletic coaches, personal trainers, Structural Integration body workers and massage therapists have a wealth of knowledge that your garden variety primary care physician may not be able to offer. If you want to condition the body, go to the folks who have made this area of knowledge their life's work and passion.

If you have struggled throughout your life with postural problems, find it hard to sit up from your bones (so-to-speak) with out feeling pain in your shoulders or spine, if you get fatigued easily, or find that your head is too far in front of your body (commonly known as: "forward head posture") a series of sessions with a Structural Integration Practitioner can help you shift out of chronic postural discomfort. Often times it is lack of muscle strength that is the cause of this weakness in the spine but if it is coupled with postural strain, you may need some more help.

Structural Integration is a hands on therapy that works specifically to get the glue out of your fascia and muscles. The method helps you learn again how to flex and extend through your back, front, sides and limbs, and lays the ground work for building strength around your spine, shoulder and hip girdles with more ease. Some times these soft tissue aberrations can bring a great deal of pain and frustration when starting a new routine of movement and getting a little hands-on help can restore your ability to move effectively and avoid injury. Not to mention most of the Structural Integration folks out there are very passionate about the body and can be a great resource in a myriad of ways. Take advantage of their natural love for health and wellness, ask questions, and enjoy the well spring of knowledge they love to share.

For trained manual therapy practitioners in your area all of these websites have information about each method with a data base to connect you with therapists all over the world.

Manual Therapy

The Rolf Institute: www.rolf.org/about
Kinesis Myofascial Integration: www.anatomytrains.com/at/kmi/
Hellerwork: www.hellerwork.com/
The St John Pain Treatment Center: www.stjohn-clarkptc.com/

Movement Re-Education

Hanna Somatics: www.hannasomatics.com/
Feldenkrais Method: www.feldenkrais.com/
Alexander Technique: www.amsatonline.org

Start Today

Start with a gentle restorative stretch class, a water aerobics class or spinning class for no impact options. Talk to your massage therapist, or physical therapist and find the right program for you. Most health insurance covers physical therapy which can be a really good place to start. For those of you who are in decent shape and just want to lose a few pounds, change things up to avoid boredom or if you are simply ready to challenge yourself, I am cheering for you from afar! Once you hit a certain level of fitness you may just want to maintain it which is great, but you may want to keep at it and see what else you are made of. Love it all! Any level at any time it is all good, really, really good. I am smiling inside at the thought of it. All of us out there stretching and moving and breathing and enhancing the life force given to us as human beings. There is tremendous personal power that is restored when we feel physically strong and capable.

There are dvd's by the truck loads that offer variety for an inexpensive home workout. Free phone apps with yoga, stretching and strength routines, friends who would love to go for a walk, hike, swim or run with you. Depending on your level of fitness you can start today with something—just get moving. A brisk walk is a great place to start and costs you nothing but a sturdy pair of comfortable shoes, or a pair of sneakers and a can-do attitude. Try a good roll on the floor or a hoof or two up the stairs at work instead of taking the elevator. Park your car at the very farthest parking spot at the store and have a good brisk walk to the door. Do some jumping jacks in your living room, spin in circles in your back yard or the park, go for a bike ride, jump in the town lake and do the doggie paddle. At first it doesn't matter *what* you do as much as it matters *that* you do. Move your body and break the habit of putting it off another minute. Just start, the rest will come, but very often it is the act of just getting started that we avoid. Again if you have a disk injury, or neck or knee injuries get some guidance and choose no impact things like swimming, biking and gentle stretching. If you are sound in your joints get a little more adventurous! Jump on a trampoline, fun, fun, fun, it reminds me of childhood, it reminds me that getting older does not have to mean losing the childlike enjoyment of flying through the air and bouncing up and down. Not to mention it is fabulous for the lymphatic system to bounce like that. I memorized the song that Tigger used to sing in Winnie The Pooh just for my trampoline time. Jumping up and down will make you giggle like mad especially if you can find a child to get on the trampoline with you, they love to laugh and it is so good for us to laugh more and have fun. Of course with any fitness routine, do a gentle warm up before you start. Roll your shoulders and your head and make some circles with your hips. Do a few squats, reach in all directions and mimic a slower form of what ever kind of exercise you are going to do. If it is swimming, do some air crawls, or air doggie paddle, if it is trampoline gently hop up and down for a few minutes. Roll out your ankles, squeeze your shoulder blades together do some standing twists and warm up a bit before you begin, but I beg of you to begin, begin right now in fact.

Chapter Highlights and Suggestions

Movement is medicine! Besides the weight loss and mood enhancing effects, moving the body is essential to keep all systems working properly. Movement keeps the respiratory, eliminatory and lymphatic systems strong and flowing. We all know the strengthening effects movement has on the cardiovascular system and of course we know it makes muscles, tendons and bones strong. If your doctors are not telling you to move more, you need different doctors, because movement is medicine, period.

- Enjoy being in physical form it is one of life's greatest pleasures!

- Soft tissues (ie: muscles, tendons, skin, organ tissue etc..) are adaptable and resilient you can get stronger and more flexible at almost any age.

- Heed your posture, if you have suffered from spinal weakness and poor posture for a long time seek professional help. See the links above to find a practitioner.

- Stiffness does not need to be a permanent state. You may need manual help. Try physical therapy, fitness coaching, massage, Structural Integration etc…refer to links above. PT is very often covered under insurance if you are short on funds.

- If you think you do not "like" exercise perhaps you just haven't found the right kind for you. There are hundreds of ways to move your body. Pumping iron at the gym is not your only option. Walk, bike, swim, jumping jacks, twirling in circles, trampoline, hiking, rowing, yoga, a dance class, or a gentle stretch class. Rent a dvd from your local library.

Try a free download. Try a few things, don't give up! Recruit a fitness buddy! No excuses!

- Try this site for free classes and fitness tracking: fitsync.com

- Or this site to track your progress: myfitnesspal.com

Touch the Earth

"My mom used to say; every day that goes by that you don't touch the earth, you are not really alive"

—*Elizabeth Gilbert*

Human beings are still dwelling in basically the same physical bodies that we evolved into hundreds of thousands of years ago. In evolutionary terms the conditions in which we now find ourselves living are relatively new given that our early ancestors trace back between about two to four hundred thousand years ago. Which means that for hundreds of thousands of years the physical human structure and physiology lived in much closer communion with the earth. Up until several hundred years ago (a very short time evolutionarily speaking) most humans lived in huts, tee pees, yurts, caves and mud structures which allowed for greater interaction with the totality of forces designed to keep us inherently strong and balanced. The home was for eating and sleeping while most time was spent out doors, hunting, gathering, fishing, and roaming about. We migrated with the seasons, we roamed far and wide powered by our limbs while we hunted and gathered our food. The passage of seasons and the rising and setting of the sun set our internal clocks. You could say that homo sapiens evolved infused by the elements and in fact I'd go as far to say we evolved as expressions of the earth from which we sprang. Is our blood not flowing through similar arterial byways like rivers flow through the landscapes etched into the earth? The internal bronchi of our lungs is not unlike the branches of trees that help cleanse the very air we breathe. The process of soil decomposing organic matter into itself is not so very different from what happens in the human digestive system. The micro bacteria in the gut decomposes food in much the same manner as the organisms in healthy soil in order to extract vital nutrients from our food. Even the organizing principle of the earth's electromagnetic field exerts an influence upon all living things, and we are still as bound to these forces in our own bodily rhythms as we ever have been.

Natural Law

There are laws at play upon this earth that if violated, come with consequences. As a culture it seems to me we are living those consequences. The conditions that come with such a fundamental disconnection from the earth happened so gradually that some of us are in a state of amnesia about what we've even lost. In fact, we have come to believe that a substantial loss of drive, inspiration and vigor at forty years old is a normal part of aging. All too often I hear people in their forties telling me they are "getting old." Their joints hurt, they have indigestion, their hair is falling out and they have no energy. These are among just a few of the symptoms people report. There also may be a vague sense that something is not right, that something is missing. Forty years old is far too young to feel so old. With the comforts, and advancements in our society we should not claim that aging has taken us in midlife. If you feel old, tired and worn out at forty years old, you are worn out before your time and that is not normal.

Plenty of us come to conclusions about the internal longing and loss of spark that hits in midlife, many have done their part to share what they've learned about these myths of our culture. Countless authors are teaching, writing and blogging about this void that we all run about trying to fill from the outside. Self help books, health and wellness books, Buddhist and secular scholars, thinkers and teachers all explaining to us that we cannot fill this thing up with stuff from the outside. Food addiction, drug addiction, alcoholism, shopping frenzies, addiction to social media and the internet and even procrastination all point to that spark which is missing. We try to fill ourselves up from the outside even for a short time, only to find that none of those things can fill us up for very long. Rest assured the craving will rise again and need to be filled. Of course everyone is so exhausted by all that consumption, the things we ingest to fill ourselves up are wearing away our hearts, livers, gallbladders, colons and stomach linings. Not to mention helping us to age prematurely and spend our golden years too run down and sick to enjoy retirement. Acceptance of the idea that this kind of premature aging is normal has been challenged by plenty of people and I applaud them. I do not believe that aging this way is normal. Many of us would feel our life force return if we immerse ourselves in the elemental forces of the earth. The earth, sun, wind, and water have restorative effects upon the human system, yet far too many people are spending too much time sheltered from the elements. This my friends needs to change!

Go Into the Light

What is to be done about this massive disconnection and early weakening of health? Where do we begin? How can we make every day changes to slowly draw ourselves back to the natural order humans were designed to live in? In part the cure is in the earth, in each of us reconnecting to the soil, the elements, the seasons, and the light. Let us start with the sun. That luminous, resonating orb in the sky that never fails to rise and nourish life upon this planet. It has only been since the early 1900s that the majority of homes where rigged for electricity and at first electricity was used sparingly due to the cost that private electricity companies charged for what was then a luxury. Compare that to the two hundred and fifty-thousand more years spent relying upon the light of the sun, moon, fire and candlelight that brought us through our days and nights. Over a short span of time we are increasingly strung to the light switch, computer screen, phone and television well beyond our biological preferences. Our sleep wake / cycles are now largely dictated by artificial lighting instead of the rising and setting of the sun and the increasing reports of sleep disorders has followed right along with it. Our flesh, blood, organs and bones developed in direct relation to the environment within which our very lives depended and we were meant to be maintained by that which created and nurtured us.

In evolutionary terms many hundreds of years is a short amount of time to expect such an ancient system to adapt to extreme disconnection from the cycles all other species on this planet adhere to. We humans are increasingly dwelling in ever more fortified homes, and spending more time inside of them than we ever have. We go from the controlled environment of heated and air conditioned homes to heated and air conditioned cars and offices. Our sun starved skin is bereft of proper amounts of vitamin D to the point where it is now standard practice for a doctor to prescribe high doses of vitamin D to a majority of patients from October to May. We've contributed to this lack of vital sunshine due to the time we do have in sunlight being spent slathered over with SPF 50 sunscreens in fear of skin cancer. There is a difference between covering yourself with baby oil while sitting on the beach at high noon every day, and allowing a reasonable amount of sun light to be absorbed into your skin every day. It is not only the skin that drinks in the light of the sun but the neural pathways from the retinas send sunlight to parts of the brain, helping to put many of our physiological processes on a 24 hour cycle. Insufficient natural light exposure can leave us with a variety of organic imbalances that effect mood, sleep, energy and vitamin D levels. Bruce Hollis, a leading vitamin D researcher at the Medical University of South Carolina reports a growing body of evidence suggesting that insufficient amounts of sunshine raise your risk of cancer, increase susceptibility to heart attack, type 1 and 2 diabetes, multiple sclerosis, arthritis, and osteoporosis.[22] So don't be afraid to get a bit of sun on your skin, in moderation of course. Those with very fair skin, moles or family history of skin cancer must be sure not to allow their skin to burn. For light skinned folks, experiment with sun screen to find the number that will allow some absorption of sunlight without allowing you to burn.

The Electromagnetic Field of the Earth

In the modern world our bodies are increasingly vulnerable to electrical interference from electromagnetic communications emanating from countless sources. Clint Ober, a telecommunications professional from Montana, has been involved in the research that brought the "Earthing Movement" forth to show us just what happens to the human body when it has been soaked in electrical currents over time without being grounded upon the earth. Increasingly, evidence confirms that the human body, with loss of ground contact, will operate in a bio-electrically stressed state. This groundless state has amplified a variety of distressing symptoms and thrown people into a state of chaos through a disruption of sufficient electrons that the human body needs to run optimally.

For example, it is common knowledge that people who develop and work with software chips must wear a grounding wire so as not to build up static on their body which can crash their project. The effect of electromagnetic fields upon the body from electrical interference

---

[22] Pludowski P, Holick MF, Pilz S, Wagner CL, Hollis BW, Grant WB, Shoenfeld Y, Lerchbaum E, Llewellyn DJ, Kienreich K, Soni M. Vitamin D effects on musculoskeletal health, immunity, autoimmunity, cardiovascular disease, cancer, fertility, pregnancy, dementia and mortality-A review of recent evidence. Autoimmun Rev. 2013 Aug; 12(10):976-89.

is real. We can't see it of course but for about twenty dollars you can go into Radio Shack and purchase a low voltage electronic meter that will show you how electrical currents interact with the human system. Every thing from lamps, hair dryers, bedside clocks and phone chargers deliver a surface charge to your body and have the potential to disrupt your metabolic system. Home appliances have a built in grounding wire as do computers, so what we are more in need of dealing with is the actual current coming off the electrical system of our homes and offices. The electricity humming away behind your walls has the ability to create electromagnetic noise which interacts with the body especially while sleeping, as many of us push our beds right up against the wall. So all night you are being bathed in electricity, which sends static and noise into your body all night while you sleep. According to Clint Ober and his research team, we should have at least the feet, uncovered, on the earth for a bit of time every day to remain balanced and grounded and to counteract the electrical currents we are exposed to every day.

The effect of the earth upon living systems cannot be underestimated. Studies have shown that connection to the earth generates a powerful and positive shift in the electrical state of the body. In fact being grounded upon the earth restores the self-healing and self-regulating mechanisms we've been naturally endowed with.[23] Connection to the earth allows a transfer of electrons (the earth's natural, subtle energy) into the body which has been shown to neutralize free radical damage caused by inflammation! If that isn't inspiration to get some bare-skin-earth-time every day I don't know what is.

Taken from the "Earthing Institute's" web site:

> *"The research indicates that Earthing transfers negatively charged free electrons into the body that are present in a virtually limitless and continuously renewed supply on the surface of the*

---

23 Chevalier and Sinatra—Grounding and Improved Autonomic Tone Integrative Medicine • Vol. 10, No. 3 • Jun/Jul 2011 17

> Earth. The existence of this unseen electron "reservoir" has been established by science. Maintaining contact with the ground allows your body to naturally receive and become charged with these electrons. When thus "grounded," any electron deficiencies and free radical excesses in the body are corrected. A natural electrical state is restored."

I find it sort of disturbing that we've had to coin a name for this lack of being on the earth. We've had to study the topic, do research upon it, and then prove the theory through research papers, books and videos. Walking bare foot upon the earth was the most natural and human thing to do not so very long ago. Now we have given it a name, we have diagnosed things that happen to us when we have become disconnected from the earth. How did we get here? How can we have become so disconnected from what we are, that we've had to start a movement with science to prove that human beings suffer when they remove themselves from the earth? We must stop this madness and remember who and what we are and where we came from.

Bring on the Bacteria!

There are other reasons to get earthy as well. We are now seeing research that the microflora of the gut react poorly when under exposed to the microbes in healthy soil. That's right—we are too clean. We have washed our hands with anti bacterial soap a few too many times. We have eaten too many antibiotics. We have killed off the balance of good and bad bacteria. Only the strongest and nastiest varieties survive and go on to birth super bugs that have ravaged across the world with few known cures. These bugs are serious. They are strong and some are unstoppable. Bacteria just *is*. We must make friends with our bacteria. Even after washing your hands, within hours the unique micro bacteria, specific to you, will begin to repopulate. So killing them is not going to happen, they are here to stay and they are an important part of our genetic makeup and immune system designed to protect us if proper balance of bacteria is maintained. The use of antibacterial gels, soaps and sprays will disrupt the balance of good and bad bacteria on the surface of your skin (or counter, or shopping cart, or baby seat etc..) and leave you more vulnerable to infection by inhospitable varieties of bacteria. We must accept that bacteria are here among us, and allow them to be. It seems far wiser to work with this by way of increasing healthy bacteria and then let those healthy varieties do their job at maintaining immunity and symbiosis with the infectious disease promoting bacteria.

The American Gut Project is doing some wonderful work to bring the importance of the flora in our guts to the forefront.[24] The study is analyzing swabs from participants to explore the relationship between gut microbes and health. A team of experts on the micro biome in human disease susceptibility and evolution will do the sequencing and analyzing of the samples, and then send the participants the results. Michael Polan, my favorite food guru, has been a vocal participant in the study. He has spoken and written about the results of his test in a most entertaining way. In an article for the New York Times called, *"Some of My Best Friends Are Germs,"* he writes: *"Our resident microbes also appear to play a critical role in training and modulating our immune system, helping it to accurately distinguish between friend and foe and not go nuts on, well, nuts and all sorts of other potential allergens. Some researchers believe that the alarming increase in autoimmune diseases in the West may owe to a disruption in the ancient relationship between our bodies and their "old friends"—the microbial symbionts with whom we co-evolved."*

That anti bacterial squirty stuff at the door to every grocery store? Forget it! Let the balance of bacteria be restored I say! Get outside and play in the dirt, touch things others have touched it's okay! When you come home simply wash with good old fashioned soap and water, it will get you clean and leave the bugs to battle things out in the way

---

24 americangut.org

they were meant to. The germ based Louis Pasteur disease model is now being challenged and we would do well to listen to the research. In another study co-led by researchers at the Universitat de València, the evidence that antibiotics produce changes in the microbial and metabolic patterns of the gut was pretty clear.[25] The study analyzed the bacteria, genes, enzymes and molecules that form the gut microbiota of patients treated with antibiotics. In the end the study suggested that the gut microbiota of people who have taken repeated doses of antibiotics end up with less of an ability to absorb iron and digest certain foods. The study also showed that an abundance of healthy bacteria could be responsible for improving the interconnection between the liver and colon and increase the production of bile acids and hormones needed for proper digestion and absorption of nutrients. So go ahead, get a little earthy, it's good for you!

Our Sedentary Lives

Our bipedal structures evolved for thousands of years walking many miles a day but now we sit at desks, and in cars for far too much time and walk an almost imperceptible amount of time compared to our ancient and not so ancient ancestors. According to the Agency for Healthcare Research and Quality between sixty and eighty percent of us will need treatment for back pain and these numbers have increased as we have become a more sedentary society. With each passing year we see more and more reports of how detrimental sitting is to our health. According to Dr Craig Liebenson director of L.A. Sports & Spine a pain management and rehabilitation center, most low back injuries are not the result of a single exposure to a high magnitude force to the spine but instead a cumulative series of events stemming from repeated small load traumas upon the spine and excessive sitting contributes more than we may realize. Low back and bio mechanics specialist and

---

25 Asociación RUVID (2013, January 9). Effects of antibiotics on gut flora analyzed. *ScienceDaily*.

author Professor Stuart McGill of The University of Waterloo reports that there is no question that excessive loading can lead to back injury, but instability at low loads is also possible and problematic.[26] [27] For example, it is possible to damage the passive tissues of the back while bending down and picking up a pencil, or sneezing, if sufficient stability of the lumbar spine is not maintained. An equal balance of both strength and flexibility can help protect the spine and getting up for a frequent walk, has clearly been shown to protect the back from the cumulative effects of sitting.

James Levine a research fellow at the Mayo Clinic has gone so far as to say that, "sitting is killing us."[28] According to the Alliance for Natural Health, sitting too much is not the same as exercising too little. They do completely different things to the body. Standing requires metabolic activity that uses lipase enzymes which grab fat and cholesterol from the blood, burning the fat into energy while shifting the cholesterol from LDL (the disease producing kind) to HDL (the disease prevention kind). When you sit, muscles are relaxed, and enzyme activity drops an alarming ninety percent, leaving fat to accumulate in the bloodstream and within a couple hours of sitting, healthy cholesterol drops by twenty percent. The trend of using stand-up desks is gaining popularity as this new research informs us that our lack of regard for our evolutionary imprint is weakening our spines to say the least. All of these deviations from our evolutionary legacy have happened in a relative blink of an eye. Thousands of years of obeying natural law has been trumped by an almost entirely simulated environment in a few hundred years.

---

26 Ikeda*, D., McGill, S.M. (2012) Can altering motions, postures and loads provide immediate low back pain relief: A study of four cases investigating spine load, posture and stability. SPINE. 37 (23): E1469-E1475
27 McGill, S.M. (2002). Low Back Disorders: Evidence- based prevention and rehabilitation. Champaign, Ill.: Human Kinetics.
28 Levine JA, et al. Move a Little, Lose a Lot. New York, N.Y.: Crown Publishing Group; 2009:26.

The Good News

We have more information at our disposal than ever before, more devices, and apps, and down loadable books, lectures, classes and papers than a person could ever possibly absorb. If used in moderation with a sprinkle of discernment these tools can be a tremendous asset, enriching our lives in a myriad of useful ways. We can no longer claim ignorance about what supports health and what does not. We can obtain information with a few minutes of surfing the internet if we are interested. We no longer have the luxury of claiming ignorance that smoking is bad for our health, that eating fake food sprayed with chemicals does not carry consequences for not only farmers, but the soil, rivers, streams, animal life and ultimately for the end user eating it. We know that the climate change is upon us. We know humans are a primary influence in this imbalance. With this knowing, comes a certain amount of personal responsibility to alter our behavior to reflect our increased understanding of the connectedness of our actions to the larger web of life. So even with the increasing pull towards sitting at your computer without a break all day, eating those fast and readily available processed foods, staying up too late staring at unnatural lights, not moving your body enough and entertaining destructive thoughts, perhaps armed with information we can become inspired to reconnect more often to those things that support health and well being. That is my utmost hope. Not everyone will embrace the incoming data steering us away from the path we are on, but I do feel that many of us will, and it is in those who embrace this shift that our hope now lays.

So what does that mean in terms of good news? It means that although we have a health epidemic due to faulty life style habits, with just a handful of adjustments we can begin the slow process of turning the ship around. There are many small things that will add up if you begin with a few life affirming habits. Life is drawn to life, so you may find that your small efforts will begin to accumulate and in time your life affirming activities will become like compounding interest in your retirement account. With each person who becomes inspired to reconnect to their ancient birth right of health and vitality the planet moves closer to restoration as well.

> *"Ultimately, in evolutionary terms in spite of how it culturally appears you do not belong to you [alone or even mostly]. You belong to the universe."*
>
> —*Buckminster Fuller.*

Chapter Highlights and Suggestions

- Garden plot anyone? Mud puddle play with your kids? Go to the beach and run the sand through your fingers and toes? Allow the earth to touch your bare skin any time, and anywhere.

- Get dirty, wash with soap, leave the anti bacterial stuff alone.

- Get ten or fifteen minutes of sunlight on your skin every day! Unless you are outside for long periods, at mid day in the heat of summer, use sunscreen sparingly and allow those fifteen minutes to be sunscreen free sun time. High elevation is different of course, as are places close to the equator. Light skinned folks use common sense so you don't burn.

- Put your bare feet, or hands or back etc on the earth every day. The earth will generously donate electrons into your body which will help reduce inflammation and reset your internal electrical system.

- Read the book *Earthing* by Clinton Ober, Steven Sinatra and Martin Zucker or visit the Earthing Institute web site for more info on this: www.earthinginstitute.net/

- Get up from your desk frequently and take a walk (outside if you can). Sit less move more!

- Move your body every day, out side if you can. Reacquaint yourself to the elements, the earth, sun, wind, and rain. Wear proper clothing and get out there! Adapting to the elements will make you an internally stronger human.

Listening to the Body

"My belief is in the blood and flesh as being wiser than the intellect."

—D.H Lawrence

Our Job as Humans

The body simply does not lie. It may endure, it may adapt, and it most certainly must remain in homeostatic balance but it will always send you truthful information about how it is functioning in the hope that you will listen and adjust accordingly. Disease and loss of our human spark happens when we ignore those signs or worse, suppress them. So at the most basic level it is our responsibility to develop, nurture and maintain an intimate relationship with this miraculous and self restorative body in which we live.

Symptoms are the way in which the body attempts to communicate information. Coughing, fever, stomach ache, bloating and heart burn, are all indications that something is not running well. Headaches, muscle pain, sinus problems, back aches, digestion problems and the like should not be ignored or suppressed but investigated, experimented with and listened to. Coughing may indicate allergy to the environment, or certain foods. Nasal cleansing is helpful for symptoms, a decongestant may help calm the symptoms down, but discovering the root cause is what really restores health. What is the cough or sinus congestion trying to tell you? Mucous is a communicator of information. Why is the immune system over reacting and is there something you can do to deal with the cause and not just the symptoms? Often times the answer is yes but the current model of medicine first and foremost moves to suppress symptoms. A wiser approach would include taking a look at the body as a connected ever evolving whole that is always working to keep itself functioning. The act of paying attention and placing meaning upon incoming information is part of our responsibility. Doctors miss things all the time, you must be aware and alert about your own flesh and blood. This is not an either/or as much as it is an *and*. It is not a call to ignore the advice of a trained health care provider but it is a call to be an active part of enhancing and supporting the help that is available. We can no longer engage in poor diet and unhealthy lifestyle choices and expect that a trip to the doctor for a pill will be enough to return us to health. It is worth the effort to consider embarking upon your own inquiry before either giving up and accepting disease, or engaging in more destructive management of symptoms via pharmaceutical suppression of them.

The Dangers of Suppressing Symptoms Through Pharmaceutical Intervention

According to The Centers for Disease Control, deaths from accidental over dose of prescription pain killers has tripled since 1990. According to Centers for Education and Research over two million accidental adverse drug reactions occur per year and about one hundred thousand of those result in death. According to the Food and Drug Administration this makes adverse drug reactions the fifth leading cause of accidental death in the United States.[29] Not to mention that more information is coming out all the time about prescription pain killers being gateway drugs to cocaine and heroin use. When the cost of prescription drugs or inability to continue to obtain a valid prescription prevents access, more people take to the streets for other alternatives.[30] Pain killers are widely used and distributed but that is not all. Depression, anxiety and sleeping pills are given out like candy, as if they are wonder cures and for some reason many doctors are not inclined to discuss lifestyle change as medicine for these disorders. Until we begin to understand that lifestyle adjustments are medicine we will continue patching people up and sending them back out into the world with their maladies well in tact. Of course there are drugs that help slow the progression of some diseases and extend lives once a disease has entered a non curable stage. Some drugs save lives, and as I've said before I am not trying to throw the baby out with the bath water. I am referring to prevention here. The medical establishment could do well to stop watching disease patterns advance only to start treating them once they are full blown. Many diseases are totally curable and through prevention many diseases can be reversed. Most prevention happens under the umbrella of lifestyle change—not pills. If it needs repeating, lifestyle change includes but is not limited to: eating real food, exercise, communing with the earth, meaningful play and work balance, sustainable stress management, engaging in positive thinking and building resiliency.

One Size Does Not Fit All

We are all constitutionally, and genetically varied yet it is an accepted practice to allow a drug into the market place for a majority of people, that has been tested and found effective for as little as thirty-three per-

---

29 National Vital Statistics Reports, Vol. 62, No. 6, p. 17 December 20, 2013
30 *Associations of Nonmedical Pain Reliever Use and Initiation of Heroin Use in the United States*, is based on data from SAMHSA's National Survey on Drug Use and Health (NSDUH), covering the period of 2002 to 2011.

cent of a control group. This means for example, that a doctor can prescribe a serotonin re-uptake inhibiting drug for treatment of depression, that worked in about three out of ten people in a control study.

Over time it became clear that treating depression with only one class of neurotransmitter drug was so ineffective for certain kinds of people that new variations targeting other brain chemicals began to be unleashed upon the public. In 2001, an advertisement for Wellbutrin, which targets both blocking the re-absorption of dopamine and norepinephrine, displayed a graph which showed the difference in efficacy between Wellbutrin and placebo is only ten percent. This information has since been removed from the Wellbutrin website but the research stands. It is hit or miss for both mental and physical health with so many medications. By taking antidepressants you could experience a host of documented side effects such as: seizures, weight gain, sleepiness, anxiety, blurred vision, headaches, tremors, insomnia, constipation and increased heart rate in addition to your depression. While the chances of it helping your depression hovers some where around ten to thirty-three percent. What about beta blockers which make the heart beat less forcefully hopefully reducing the possibility of hyper tension that leads to heart attacks? You may go to the doctor for high blood pressure and end up with drug side effects like, asthma, depression, insomnia or sexual dysfunction and these beta blocking drugs have not been shown to reduce the incidence of heart attack in people over the age of sixty. There are other ways to prevent a heart attack, of that you can be sure.

I am not advocating not going to the doctor. Heart disease and depression are serious stuff and being under the care of a doctor to know just where you stand is imperative. What I am advocating is that we can all do better in *preventing* these situations from occurring at all. That is real medicine. Not waiting and watching symptoms increase while doing nothing to reverse them. With lifestyle change we have the power to prevent certain common diseases like diabetes, heart disease, stroke, gout, Celiac's Disease, and irritable bowel syndrome. We are also seeing some movement toward more personalized drug treatments through the advancements in stem cell research and as interesting and hopeful as this is, it has been driven by decades of medication failures to eradicate lifestyle illness. People have erroneously mistaken management and suppression of symptoms via pharmaceuticals as a cure for ailments that are due to faulty life style habits. Lifestyle correction often times delivers a full cure where drugs merely mask the symptoms leaving in place the illusion that you can keep offending your bodily filtration systems through poor habits and get away with it. It is dangerous to ignore the signs because in time if you don't listen, something greater will have to occur, sometimes that something greater is an irreversible disease that will seriously interrupt your life and eventually lead to a needlessly premature death.

Medication is not the cure for bad choices....better choices are.

Scientific Advancements

That being said, we are moving forward in a more intelligent administration of medication. Certain conditions can be well treated when the mystery of the cause has been revealed. In some cases a more subtle deficiency that is organic in nature can be cured with just the right substance. The National Institute of Health scientists have made significant progress toward uncovering the medical potential of stem cells and have developed new tools for genome sequencing. Scientists are learning more about how genes affect our health, and how a genetic approach can help doctors customize treatments and prevention strategies for individual patients. I love the prevention part! It is becoming more evident that research into prevention is where we will get the most bang for our buck. It is still a new area of research but it is exciting. One of the most exciting things that has been discovered through gene research is epigenetics.

Epigenetics

Epigenetics is the study of changes in genes which are *not* caused by changes in the DNA alone. Unlike simple *genetic* changes to our DNA, *epigenetics* research has revealed that very often the way genes react have other causes than just pure family history. Our living environment, stress responses, diet, exercise, emotional states etc, are now scientifically proven to influence patterns of disease as are other subtle causes of organic or genetic deficiency.[31] The good news is that we can either program our genes to express disease, or program them to express health. You may have the propensity for stroke, heart attack or diabetes in your family but those genes do not have to condemn you to those fates.

Unlike behavior or stress, diet is more easily studied when it comes to epigenetics. The nutrients we extract from food enter metabolic pathways where they are altered into elements the body can use, as are chemicals and other irritants that can damage DNA and turn on disease promoting chain reactions. For example, The University of Utah has done studies that have shown that deficiency of methyl-donating folate or choline during pregnancy or early postnatal development causes certain regions of the genome of the fetus to be under-methylated for life. It may mean the person with these genetic predispositions will need to take good sources of folate and choline daily to correct and support this inherent deficiency. Without enough folic acid anemia could be a lifelong problem that can get passed into the next generation. Uncovering these genetic alterations in DNA can offer targeted treatment plans to increase the needed nutrient specific to each of us to bring our bodies into stronger states of wellness. This kind of medicine holds great promise, and is a kind of deep listening. Instead of throwing a substance into the body and hoping that it sticks, we are evolving towards gathering the necessary information to administer medicine

---

31   McGowan P.O., Meaney M.J., Szyf M. (2008). Diet and the epigenetic (re)programming of phenotypic differences in behavior. Brain Research, 1237: 12-24

in a more intelligent manner. In addition to our own observations and listening, the body can be brought back to health when it receives just what it needs to function best. So let us not ignore symptoms. Listen to those symptoms, consider the intelligence behind them, and then enter into a partnership with your body and make the adjustments in lifestyle to correct them at the root cause.

Chapter Highlights and Suggestions

- The body never lies! We must listen and respond when it is speaking to us via symptoms.

- Medications can only be tested so much, are often only effective in a small percentage of people and almost all of them have harmful side effects.

- Suppression of symptoms is NOT a cure do not be mistaken in this!

- Symptoms are a call for a correction of an offending habit not a call for a straight jacket for the symptoms.

- Embark on your own experiments to understand your symptoms. For example: if you are suffering from chronic migraines try eliminating common triggers like red wine, sugars, food chemicals, smoking and gluten.

- Consider inquiring with your doctor for gene specific tests for just the right correction for you.

- Educate yourself about Functional Medicine at www.functionalmedicine.org/ with this kind of primary care your physician will work to find the real cause of illness and partner with you to integrate the corrections needed into your life.

For Example:

- Maybe genetically you do not absorb calcium that well and that is why you have early thinning of bone. Calcium that is absorbed easier than tablets (such as sub lingual or liquid varieties) and higher doses of calcium may correct the problem more completely than something like "Forteo" (the accepted norm for bone density loss which can cause bone cancer if taken for more than two years) additionally adding weight bearing exercise can help prevent further bone loss.

- Perhaps you are missing enzymes that break down dairy and that is why you have excess mucous. Taking a digestive enzyme may eradicate the problem where suppressing the symptoms would make the condition worse over time. Cutting back on dairy to rest your system may diminish the discomfort while adding an enzyme targeted towards helping digest dairy could help your body heal and the mucous may subside. Perhaps this could even allow you to have small amounts of dairy, symptom free, again over time.

- Perhaps you have developed sensitivity to gluten and instead of understanding this you take a laxative in an attempt to relieve belly bloating or antacids to suppress indigestion but keep eating pasta and bread etc.. All the while your ability to absorb nutrition declines, the sensors in your colon are further damaged and you end up giving yourself full blown Celiac's Disease. If caught early enough and treated with eliminating gluten from the diet you can prevent the full expression of the disease from manifesting.

Going Unplugged

"What information consumes is rather obvious: it consumes the attention of its recipients. Hence a wealth of information creates a poverty of attention"

—*Herbert Simon*

A new global study of university students by the International Center for Media & the Public Agenda (ICMPA) asked one thousand college students from various countries to go twenty-four hours without their media devices. The students were then asked to report on the experience. They expressed a variety of distressing feelings from the experiment like this report from a student of the USA: "*I was itching, like a crackhead, because I could not use my phone.*" A student from Argentina observed: "*Sometimes I felt 'dead,'*" and a student from Slovakia offered: "*I felt sad, lonely and depressed.*"

Also of note was a realization that cyber connection was an integral part of their personal identities. "*I literally didn't know what to do with myself,*" said one student from the UK, and another shared about every day necessities being boring: "*Going down to the kitchen to pointlessly look in the cupboards became a regular routine, as did getting a drink."* Almost all of the subjects quickly became bored and lost interest in the alternative activities they did try. Some students became bored within a few hours; others in even less time than that. Said one student from China: *"After fifteen minutes without using media, my sole feeling about this can be expressed in one word: boring."* A student from Mexico stated: *"It was an unpleasant surprise to realize that I am in a state of constant distraction, as if my real life and my virtual life were coexisting in different planes, but in equal time."* The study also asked students to report about times when they did not stick with the experiment and it turned out that many were simply not able to complete the 24 hour time period without their devices. Many using words like: "addiction" and "withdrawal."

Addiction is defined in Webster's Dictionary as a compulsive need for and use of a habit-forming substance (or activity) characterized by tolerance and by well-defined physiological symptoms upon withdrawal; and persistent compulsive use of a substance known by the user to be harmful. I am pretty sure we can say any one walking around with their phone in their pocket or hand all day who compulsively checks Twitter, Facebook, emails, texts and messages and cannot function or find meaning in life without it, is addicted. Device addiction is accompanied by a wide range and variety of harmful effects that can be seen on the road, in the stores, in schools, at home and in the work place. How can people pay adequate attention as they move through their day when they are so preoccupied with what is inside those devices? What is happening to us? It's like we don't see each other any more, we don't care to talk anymore, we would rather text or leave a Facebook message. With people de-humanizing each other from the autonomous nature of communicating not in person, but with short quick word bytes on the phone or via email, we are seeing bullying in schools that has led to countless suicides in teen and pre-teen students. In a study done by Dalhousie University in Halifax that analyzed forty-one cases of suicide with a cyber bullying component, social networking sites were used in forty-eight percent of all the suicide cases, while messaging (text, pictures or video) were used in twenty-five percent of the cases.[32] Being a teenager is hard enough without adding this sort of bullying to the mix.

Where Does the Time Go?

Have you ever found yourself asking, "where did the last hour go?" when lingering in internet social networks? Does time seem to slip away as you notice that another day has gone by and you have not accomplished what you wanted to? Social media is like a drug; it takes only short term exposure and we can't help but want more. There are many things about this phenomenon that will have long term consequences for both the user and society as a whole and we have gone far beyond reversing this trend. These devices are here to stay and as of this moment it does not appear that any discretion is being exercised in terms of just how much time people are submerged in this alternate reality. Why does it matter you may ask? Everyone is doing it and it is just the way people interact now. Have we really considered the consequences of this level of distraction and immersion in the cyber world and is it really all that troubling? I believe the answer if you think on it for a time is, *yes*. There are a variety of studies appearing that track the harmful societal trends emerging directly from the overuse of digital devices such as, decreased memory and concentration skills, lack of interest in the real world, eye strain, wrist pain, headaches, neck tension, anxiety, depression, frustration, lack of patience, lack of empathy towards others, anger, and procrastination. Just like any other addictive substance or activity, these cultural device dependent movements are effecting us.

We see instant gratification becoming an entitlement that creates

---

32   http://www.cbc.ca/news/technology/story/2012/10/19/cyberbullying-suicide-study.html

impatience, anger and frustration if any task takes more than a few minutes or involves the need for patience and calm. I would submit that the general human character has taken a hit in all of this and we are becoming the sort of people none of us want to become. Texting while driving has become another rampant occurrence of late which has created a whole new atmosphere on the roads. It never ceases to astonish me when I glance over at the car next to me and the driver is studiously focused upon their lap with an occasional glance at the road, or the phone is actually perched upon the dash board with one hand texting and the other on the wheel. Turn signals have become a relic of the past, of course, because there is no free hand for such activities. Drivers taking sudden unannounced turns, cutting other drivers off, and aggressive horn honking have taken over the roads as well as very little personal responsibility when the aggressive or half present driver has violated the rules of the road. In fact often you will be the lucky recipient of the middle finger salute if you dare to object to someone who has only half an eye and a quarter of their attention on the road. We are in a whole different world now. Personally I think it is a dangerous trend that further distances us from each other as human beings and creates a chaotic society of self absorbed and distant people. A collective denial has swept through our nation as we are compulsively drawn further into our electronic devices instead of engaging fully with each other and the real world.

Of the quotes from the ICMPA study that struck me the hardest was the lack of these students being able to engage in the real world in the absence of their devices. How empty things were for them was striking, as if they were just bodies going through the motions of life. Without their external "media brains" they could not think for themselves or find anything meaningful to do or experience out there in the real world. They became sort of like zombies. Life became boring and lost meaning for them. There is nothing boring about the real world. I enjoy tinkering in my flower beds, reading a book, going for a walk, lunch or sharing a meal with friends, practicing guitar or mandolin, writing in my journal and puttering about in the kitchen, just as I always have. The phone is around some where, but it is not what I am thinking about until it rings. The first snow is still magical, spring trees in bloom never cease to bring a smile to my face, and going for a run or bike ride in the sun or the rain for that matter, has a renewing effect upon the deepest parts of my psyche. How on earth could this big, messy, beautiful world be boring? To think that without a flashing, beeping phone nearby, all of these daily happenings of life would become empty and meaningless is disturbing. For the students in that study it meant that individual thoughts, ideas and real world interaction were basically non-existent. College age adults walking about like empty shells, with no original thoughts, feelings or ideas being generated on their own. Without a device in their hands they felt they had "too much time" and they could not find a single thing to do that would bring them joy or satisfaction. How many people yearn for more time? There is not enough hours in the day to get things done, I hear this quite a bit and yet when faced with all this free time without devices people were bored and lost. They have become slaves to their phones and computers. Their days being dictated by who calls, who texts, and who "likes" their Facebook post and follows a Twitter feed. With many of these interactions being of a highly mundane subject matter and only offering the illusion of real intimate human connection. This is not isolated to college students either, an alarming number of people of all ages go through every day of their lives with their attention drawn into a virtual world with only fragments of themselves truly engaged, responding, thinking and feeling the actual world.

In his books and lectures Nicholas Carr offers compelling evidence regarding what the dark side of the digital age is doing to our brains. Carr is a best selling author and Pulitzer Prize nominee who has written several books on Information Technology. One of which is called, *The Shallows: What the Internet is Doing to Our Brains.* He explains how books helped us to focus our attention which promoted deep and creative thought. Conversely however, the internet and social media encourages rapid and distracted samples of information from many sources. In today's world, speed and efficiency are king. Consumption has become the law of the land under this king, and now the cyber world is remaking us in its own image. We are becoming ever more efficient at scanning and skimming, but we are losing our capacity for concentration, contemplation, and self reflection. I see it every day, aggressive social interaction where people have little or no regard for how they are affecting the world around them. Where just a little reflection and pause may bring us back to a place of realizing that our distracted presence has an impact on the people around us. When we walk around with our faces stuffed into phones we are perhaps unknowingly being a bit like Mister Magoo! We walk out into parking lots and streets with hardly a glance at traffic, we bump into people, ignore people, and have a general lack of regard for the real world activities that continue to go on all around us as we are pinned to the phone. Every day I see someone talking on the phone while at a check-out line, as if that person helping at the register is a nobody. Why has this become in some way, acceptable social behavior?

Some of you may be reading this thinking I am an old fashioned stick-in-the-mud who is missing out on the wonders of virtual reality. While others of you are perhaps nodding your heads in agreement at my concerns around this issue. For those of us who spent the first twenty, thirty or more years without these gadgets, we remember and know that we can get along fine with moderate use of them, we do not seem to be as addicted as younger generations. Despite the fact that it has been proven that the instant gratification of the virtual world is indeed addictive especially to the young developing brain.[33] It may be easier for those of us raised without them to have some level of self control. So far I manage just fine with a regular cell phone and lap top, checking email a few times a day. I do a fair share of scheduling sessions with my clients via email and text, and I am a music junkie who most

---

33   Wilhem Hofman, Baumeister, R. F., Foerster, G., & Vohs, K., "Everyday temptations: An experience sampling study of desire, conflict, and self-control," *Journal of Personality and Social Psychology, 102*, 1318-1335 (2012).

definitely enjoys the portability of an iPod. I think the key words with these things are: *use in moderation*.

Free will is a dangerous thing. It is riddled with consequence. We come back to free will again here, we can make choices based on what we know about the downside of technology. I am not suggesting we all need to do away with our devices, technology can be of great value if used with some level of discretion. So that you use it, instead of it using you. This cultural shift to virtual reality could be modified so that it does not have so many people within such a tight grip. Addictions can be intercepted and shifted even if only just enough to allow people to take back a bit of their lives and stay human. I am hoping that at least a few of the participants in the aforementioned study had reason to pause and re-evaluate their dependence upon technology after they witnessed first hand the effects it had upon their sanity.

Another Opportunity for an Experiment!

I have started a little experiment with myself, it began with deactivating my Facebook account which has proven a most worthy reclamation of more time in which to complete the writing of this book, among other things. The experiment then expanded with powering down my phone for a portion of a day, once a week and I limited my internet time to a few fifteen minute intervals per day. Generally I am a hobby surfer with the occasional need to research something, book a trip, or gather information for one thing or another. Except for the months spent writing this book I have pretty much become accustomed to the limits I put on the use of my phone and computer. For those folks who are in the technology industry clearly this experiment would not work so well unless you try it on a weekend. Even half a day on a weekend could be a good start to gaining more personal freedom from those devices. An experiment like this might allow for you to explore where your own thoughts have gone off to, or to reclaim your creativity and a bit of your time.

Focus, Action and Creativity in the Cyber Age

Again I emphasize that technology can and is being used for tremendous good and for wonderful creative purposes by countless companies and highly creative people. I refer more to the trouble emerging when we use these devices as distraction and procrastination tools or in place of real human connection. If you are someone who has a bucket list, or a daily to-do list or a dream of completing a large project or creative pursuit that sits on the back burner day after day, what can be done to mitigate this habit?

In some ways the leap from having an idea to executing an idea is where many people get stuck. Ideas may fly around, but can you grab one by the tail and really engage with it long enough to see it materialize? Are you frustrated because your bucket list or important to-do list goes constantly undone as the days whiz by filled with the management of the mundane? The texts, the emails, the papers, bills, and shopping all pulling you away from that little nagging dream of creating something of real substance? Being able to stay with a thought or idea long enough to bring it into an action phase of development can be daunting if your distraction rate is high. I believe the constant allure of phones and computers has cemented this high level of distraction quite deeply into our behaviors. It is a habit ingrained over years of multitasking and skim-the-surface-living. The only one who can retrain us to stay steady and focused—is us. It is the exact opposite of the fight-or-flight response that must be exercised in order to remain calm and focused long enough to follow through on an idea or creative pursuit.

In my meditation classes I echo quite frequently that distraction just *is*. There may never be a perfect time, or a perfect place to meditate, or start your grand idea or find your purpose and create the physical manifestation of it. There will always be the allure of engaging with the myriad of distractions coming at us, whether those distractions come from our minds, the phone, the kids, or your job. These responsibilities are real, and require our attention. However, learning to trust that some of those distractions can wait for you, is a tough one. We are so well trained to jump into action at the slightest provocation, that we are no longer able to pause and wait, but it is there in the pause and in the waiting, that the space to create lives. It is there in those in-between moments that your meditative and creative state quietly waits for you to engage with it. It is you who must sit still and trust that in the space of that stillness and non-doing is all the stuff of concentration, focus and creativity. Even if at first it feels rather useless and unproductive. I am not saying the space is *it*. The space is not ultimately *it*. The space will not create the thing for you, only your direct action and will power can do that. However, the will power and creative human fire in most of us, cannot be blown into a spark without the air of space.

So if in the back of your mind you are being nagged by The Muse to write that poem or grow that garden, try sitting quietly and allowing your mind to visualize it. If you are feeling called to write that book, start or finish that business, put paint to easel, reorganize your closets or junk drawer, find some time to contemplate and consider a plan of action. If you are wanting to make that fabulous dish and share it with friends, learn a language, or a musical instrument and you cannot seem to do it, see what might happen if you sit still and wait while holding the thought of your goal in your mind until the impetus to act rises. Put your phone away, shut off your computer, and find a time when the kids are in school and you have a few moments to sit still, consider your idea, and how you can make it happen. Before anything can materialize it must first start as a thought. So dream, visualize, see it happen, behave as if this thing you hope to achieve has already begun to happen. The time to be with your creative idea may not appear magically, you may need to actively create it, demand it in fact and simply just take the time for yourself. Sitting still is not the only way to create an internal atmosphere that supports creative action and problem solving. Sometimes taking a walk in the woods, at a park or on the beach will help clear your mind of the mundane long enough for The

Muse to stop by. Try some stream of consciousness writing. What clears your mind? A bath? Laying on the floor? Yoga? A nap? Picking weeds? You decide, it doesn't matter as much *how* you do it, but *that* you do it and do it in the absence of any kind of external digital device. This requires your full attention free of distraction and free from what I like to call the "external media brain." You may begin to hear the whispers of solutions emerging, you may begin to see a clear path of first steps to take to manifest your idea but first you must create the space for the answers to speak to you. For those of you who can create under any circumstance, (I know you are out there) you may not need these practices but for those of you struggling with procrastination, or self sabotage give this a try and see if you don't begin to have a full blown relationship with the part of you that was born to create.

You may also find that your memory and patience slowly begin to improve or that ideas to develop a new skill seem more inviting. Challenging the brain with learning a new skill creates new synapses and neural plasticity that helps slow down the aging process. You may find that you enjoy the new found time that gets created when the hours once spent online are spent interacting with the real world. Take it one day at a time as they say, start with small steps that do not overwhelm and don't hurry the process, but if you can, begin to disengage from constant digital interaction. You may find that a host of irritating happenings in your life naturally clear themselves up in the process. Have a look at both the Artful Living chapter and the Meditation and Stillness chapter for more tips and ideas on these topics. For aid in the development of focus and concentration a group of neuroscientists have gotten together and created brain games based on brain plasticity. If you want to sharpen your mental skills through scientifically created brain games, check out lumosity.com. Just one more way to use the internet to build your brain power, remember, use it, don't let it use you by giving in to mindless surfing to kill time and avoid real action.

Chapter Highlights and Suggestions

- Make yourself aware of the research that shows the negative effects of media addiction on focus, concentration, productivity and long term goals.

- Consider how time management and goal setting become easier when you take time every day for your own thoughts.

- Consider honestly if you might be addicted to digital devices and inquire into the effects it is having upon your life.

- Multitasking has not been shown to increase productivity or retention of information, in fact the opposite is shown to be true.

- The real world is truly magical and has effects upon your natural rhythms. Uninterrupted time in the real world is essential to develop new ideas and creativity.

Start Small

- Let emails sit in favor of taking care of more important priorities that nurture long term goals.

- Take daily fifteen minute media breaks to start and increase by five minutes a day.

- Focus on one thing at a time and see if it increases your productivity and has calming effect upon your stress level.

- Take time in nature every single day, leave your device at home during this time.

- Notice little improvements in your concentration, memory and patience after a few weeks of focused time without your external media brain.

- Try the training program at lumosity.com to build concentration, memory, and problem solving skills.

Not Good Enough

And did you get what you wanted from this life, even so?
I did.
And what did you want?
To call myself beloved, to feel myself
beloved on the earth.

—*Raymond Carver*

The very idea that any human being, who took trillions of cells to create by the life giving forces of this universe, is not good enough—is unfathomable. If you believe you are not good enough you are hooked into a lie. If there is something consistent to note after working with people in a therapeutic setting for almost two decades, it would be that many feel they will never be good enough. We push and punish ourselves relentlessly with negative self talk and poor life style choices. Perhaps then at some point, when we are finally close to being utterly beaten down, when we are sick, depressed, over weight and lonely we may look around and ask if there is another way to live. This is the place where healing can begin. When we have simply had enough of the destructive, disease promoting habits that we've accepted for the better part of our lives we go in search of the road back to freedom and health. Good for us! Oh the road is long and winding but we must make the first step and begin because staying where we are is not an option if we want to live, I mean really live.

This belief that we are not good enough can create obstacles in every area of life. It keeps us from realizing our potential, creates guilt and shame due to that stalling grip upon starting, or finishing a project or going after a dream. Not to mention how it informs our food and life style choices and who and what we embrace as friends, partners and jobs. Those patterns that keep showing up which bring pain, sadness and frustration can be extremely difficult to change if we are operating from a place of feeling inadequate and unworthy of anything better. A variety of things attempt to cover the belief up, it hides in the shadows trying to point us in other directions for answers. It may show up as control issues, anxiety, depression, body pain, insecurity, procrastination, bullying, or jealousy etc. We try to treat those myriad of symptoms all while this fundamental belief goes unrealized, this much deeper belief that *drives* all those other self destructive patterns. The under ground, subconscious belief that: "I am not good enough" is running the show from the depths of our private internal world. We could dive into how this old, well woven fabric of a belief system begins for people but I am not a psychologist, sociologist or mental health councilor and I'm not qualified to say I have some kind of easy solution for this problem, but I can offer some of the things that have helped me alter this mindless wheel of crazy self loathing thoughts.

All the confusing messages and heart break of life can ravage our sense of well being, cloud the lens through which we view the world and bring our very existence onto question. For countless reasons and in countless ways people are doing what they can to manage the emptiness of being flawed humans. The murky under world of addiction starts here as we go about trying to fill ourselves from the outside, and do things that give us temporary feelings of relief with food, drugs, alcohol, gambling, sex, and a host of other life threatening things. If we could turn the feelings of unworthiness down a notch or two, often times many of those compulsive habits resolve enough to live a more meaningful and healthy life. Turning it down a bit can take the pressure off, the expectation that embarking upon this journey will eradicate all pain and suffering is unrealistic, but to let go of bits and pieces of it at a time will go a long way to restoring your body and mind.

If we fundamentally think we are not worth much we develop destructive lifestyle habits that can be difficult to shift. At what point does our own internal power awaken and come into play in the process of unwinding all the symptoms that lead back to this one powerful belief? How can we point to one place and say; "*that's it*!" that is where I hold my self loathing, that is what holds me back from blooming into my highest potential. It is in my belly, I better go to the belly doctor and clean this up. Then it may show up in the neck from the tension of trying to control the world, so off we go to the neck doctor to see if they might be able to help us. We feel bad about ourselves so we drink soda and eat boxes of cookies for the rush of sugar and carbohydrates. The serotonin released from the sugars might make us feel better for about an hour even though the sugar, over time destroys our ability to create serotonin. Later, feeling bloated, sick and shameful we declare we must go on a diet and get this binge eating under control. The wheel of addiction could go on and on like this. The cure could remain a mystery. If we chop ourselves all up into pieces and chase the dragons around in circles trying to slay them one by one we may end up feeling pretty frustrated. Years could go by while mental, emotional and physical health begin to decline. What if we went right to the source of what is driving us to make poor choices, could it help us grow and change in new ways? Might it help us make choices that support life and not decay and disease?

Self loathing is a system-wide phenomenon and it does not reside in a single place. We could go to fifty doctors and still there will be an endless loop of symptoms. To unleash it from the holding cells of our imaginations we must do more than talk about it or feed it pills and hope that some out side source will come and save us. This is not to say if you are in therapy and working on this issue, that you should stop. Keep at it. A qualified therapist can be a huge part of unraveling and understanding the effects of self loathing upon your life. It is not to say that the temporary therapeutic use of medication cannot be a help, but we also must do our part and not rely solely on outside sources. We can be an active participant in our own healing and come out on the other side of this feeling empowered and more whole. There are additional ways of facing and realizing how self defeating thoughts play out that are our responsibility. There is no single big solution, those days are gone, what we know about healing, and I mean systems-wide deep healing, is that it is a process. There is no magic bullet, we've exhausted that idea and it has proven time and again to be temporary and come with a host of unsavory side effects. All while the insidious effects of self loathing are allowed to remain fully operational wreaking havoc in every dimension of our lives. This belief not only lodges in our thoughts but in our cells, our fluids, our flesh, bones and blood, it is deep and it is powerful. Addressing this not only in the mind but in the body as well, is an important part of the journey to self discovery, self acceptance and a generally healthier and more content existence.

Always Do Your Best. Your best is going to change from moment to moment; it will be different when you are healthy as opposed to sick. Under any circumstance, simply do your best, and you will avoid self-judgment, self-abuse and regret.

—*Don Miguel Ruiz*

The Mind Body Connection

The mission statement at Massachusetts General Hospital's Mind

Body Medicine program started by doctor Herbert Benson has this to say about the importance of the mind body connection: *Through a "cognitive/behavioral" approach, we help patients better recognize the self-defeating thoughts, negative statements, and irrational beliefs that undermine our mood, behavior, and health.*

Mass General goes on to explain their mission further: *The Benson-Henry Institute for Mind Body Medicine is a non-profit scientific and educational organization dedicated to research, teaching, and clinical application of mind/body medicine and its integration into all areas of health.*

Oh yes, major hospitals and research centers including the National Institute of Health, which is quite literally among the largest governmental institutes charged in safe guarding our nations health, is even on the case of the mind body connection. What we think and how we perceive the world exerts a tremendous influence upon our health. What happens to the mind, happens to the body. We will take a look at the importance of bodily movement in the healing process later on in this chapter. The body/mind is real, the time has arrived for us all to realize that the mind, our thoughts, and how we perceive the world play an enormous role in our lives. I believe it is official; Life, Liberty and The Pursuit of Happiness is an inside job!

An Inside Job

In the next hour or so take some time to actually become conscious of the thoughts that play over and over in your mind. Much of the time we let these thoughts run "mindlessly" almost taking for granted that they are just there. Always, they are just there. We don't often interrupt them to examine if they are actually true or consider the effect they may be having upon our health and well being. We allow them to use us, these unconscious words running over and over, making grooves in the pathways of our body and mind. So I ask you, to take a few minutes as you go about your life in the next hour, every now and then catch a thought as it swims by and ask yourself a few questions about it: "is that true, is it kind, is it helpful, and would I say it out loud to another person?" If you suspect the thought is not true, ask yourself if you believe it and why, if you do not believe it consider the effect of allowing a lie to live inside your thoughts. If it is not kind, and not helpful consider that for a moment, are you an essentially unkind person? If not, let that sink in. If you are not an unkind person, why would you want to berate yourself with self depreciating thoughts? If you would never say those things to a friend why would you say them about yourself? Maybe this thought experiment reveals to you that you are an unkind person, do you want to be? Or are you just unkind on auto pilot because you were treated unkindly in the past? There could be pain there, you may need a qualified therapist to safely guide you back to your true nature. I don't know too many down right mean spirited babies. Most of us did not show up here on this earth angry and mean. Life can break us, but we can put ourselves back together again. Try to understand the workings of your own mind, bring the light of consciousness and truth to those thoughts. Examination is the first step toward understanding and change. The next step is simply being with the thought, with no resistance. Do not move to defend yourself or the thought. If it brings up emotion, and it is attached to a memory get yourself into therapy right away and do your best not to ignore it and shove it back down into the basement of your soul. Invite these negative thoughts to come out, into the clear light of day where they can be dealt with in the open. Just because you stuff it down does not mean it has no influence upon your life, quite the opposite.

If you would never in a million years say this thought out loud in the presence of another person allow yourself to really feel that. What would it mean if you said the thought out loud, how would it effect your relationships, would it poison them? Consider that there is hardly a difference in the effect upon your body/mind between saying it out loud in the presence of another and keeping the thought to yourself.

The poison is the same. Those negative thoughts effect your chemistry, your organs, your muscles and your hormones. Your entire intelligent, thinking, feeling self registers those thoughts, files them away, and allows them to inform your behavior and your physical health. Feel the weight of the fact that if your thoughts tend to be negative, self depreciating, and unkind you can do something about it if you first become aware the thoughts even exist. Just observe your thoughts, see if you can look at them without any story what so ever attached. No one else can see or hear this process, it is personal, so you can be totally honest with yourself here. Just because you have a thought, does not automatically make it true. Any unexamined self abusive thought is suspect and if you examine the thought and find it is not true and you would never say it out loud either about yourself or another person, I would encourage you to consider letting the thought leave. Realize it is not true. At some point when you can, even smile at it next time it runs through, (because it will keep showing up well after you get hip to it). In time you will get more aware that the thought is not actually true. If it is true, consider that and see if you can reframe it so you can turn the thought into a vehicle for change and self love. If you know you can do better, but you cannot figure out how, maybe it is time to get some help, admit that you cannot do it alone and begin to make positive changes in your life. Some times we cannot be accountable to ourselves alone and we need a mentor or guide to report to in the beginning until new habits take hold. You are worth it, of that you can be sure. The process of unhinging these unexamined beliefs takes time and effort so do your best not to set up an unrealistic expectation. Notice it, shine the light of truth on it, and let it go a million times until it no longer has a charge to it. It could take years to actualize a true letting go of those lies running in your mind and body. If you don't at least consider challenging them, two years from now you will be further degraded by them instead of well on your way to allowing them to lose their influence over you.

Reach out for support, fill your eyes and ears with life affirming words, music, books, poetry, and movies. Turn off the news and put down the fashion magazines, you are poisoning your own self, you are programming yourself with lies and misinformation. Only you can stop this madness.

How often is an act of your kindness shown to another and not to yourself? It is not indulgent to think well of yourself especially if it can make you a more effective, productive and internally content person. I am not advocating conceit, that is a different thing entirely. Thinking well of yourself does not automatically come along with thinking less of others. If we have need of anything in this war weary and violent world it is more people who are gentle, thoughtful and kind and that begins within each of us. We are often much kinder to others than we are to ourselves. The next time you buy or pick flowers for a friend, why not do the same for yourself. The next time you offer some consoling advice to an aching heart, why not offer those same words to your own aching heart. The next complimentary words you pass onto a friend, can you say those same words to yourself? Even if you don't believe them at first just go ahead and "fake it till you make it." It may not be authentic at first but if you keep at it, you will in time replace the programming from your past, which very well could be a real pack of lies, into new and more self respecting thoughts. Our thoughts are full of beliefs from the media, siblings, parents, acquaintances etc..that may have been erroneous opinions that you mistook for truth. Make new neural pathways of respect and positive thoughts for yourself, and then watch what that does to your life.

Neuroplasticity

Neuroplasticity has replaced the formerly held belief that the brain is a physiologically static organ, and explores how the brain changes throughout life. From cellular changes due to learning, to large-scale changes involved in cortical remapping in response to injury, we now know that the brain is fully capable of building new neural pathways well into adulthood.[34] In other words, the brain is pliable and adaptable. Until recently neuroscientists believed that the brain is relatively immutable after early childhood. This belief has been challenged by research revealing that many aspects of the brain remain responsive to neuronal growth into adulthood. The brain cannot build new pathways unless you, the person with the brain, exercises the neural pathways within the mind. Your thoughts are powerful, so choose the ones that will empower and strengthen you, not the ones that tear you down. No one gets to do that without your consent, not even you.

The discovery of neuroplasticity enables us to trust that our brains can change, they can expand, get stronger and embrace new ideas and thought patterns, this is hopeful news. What happens to the brain via the thoughts happens to the body and the reverse is also true. This is a call to keep learning, keep growing and challenging yourself. It is a good reason to check yourself if you find you are becoming negative in your thoughts out of habit. Research shows that optimism is not only a heritable trait but can be developed with practice and can increase quality of life and success. [35] Positive thinking is one of those things that centenarians (people who live to be one hundred years and older) around the world do whether they realize it or not. Positive thoughts have been found to be an integral component of longevity. This is not to say suppress your emotions, or deny authentic human feelings of anger, sadness and grief. The distinction between the habit of seeing the world through a distorted negative lens is not the same as facing and coping with serious feelings of pain and loss. There will be a bit more on this in the chapter on Resiliency.

---

34 Brain Plasticity and Behavior Bryan Kolb,[1] Robbin Gibb, and Terry Robinson Canadian Centre for Behavioural Neuroscience, University of Lethbridge, Lethbridge, Alberta, Canada (B.K., RG.), and Department of Psychology, University of Michigan, Ann Arbor, Michigan (T.R.)

35 Optimism, coping, and health: Assessment and implication of generalized outcome expectancies, Scheier, Micheal F,;Carver, Charles S. Health Psychology, Vol 4 (3), 1985, 219-247

Posture and Self Esteem

A strong flexible body often goes right along with a strong flexible mind. A slumped over, caved in body goes along with depression, anxiety and fear in the mind. It has been true in my body work practice that the folks who come in and slump down in the chair as we talk through their health history, suffer from some kind of anxiety and depression. During postural assessments at the start of sessions, I consider how to treat based on postural patterns that are locked into a person's physical structure. If there is internal rotation of the humeral heads (aka: caved in chest and rounded shoulders and upper back) and a forward head posture, with a tight jaw and iron-like quality to the back of the neck, I've already learned something about the person's story. Often times this person has had a life long struggle with low self esteem, depression and negative thoughts bearing down on them. It is very clear and obvious what this postural pattern means and how it expresses itself in the personality. It is the first order of business to get an understanding of the filter through which people view the world, and consider how this view has carved its way into their posture. To include and observe the quality of bodily tissues is an integral piece of healing. When a person is ready and willing to let go, accept help and take personal responsibility, things do get more hopeful. As the body changes the mind may begin to shift. If we can shift and release those stuck physical patterns a variety of unconscious beliefs begin to change. When we get that person more upright through the chest, belly and spine, bring them a more solid stance through the hips, legs and feet, soften the grip of the jaw and neck, watch out! I've seen catharsis time and time again as the muscular and nervous system energy that was being used to grip tight against the world is released and then gathered up in new ways. Tears, anger, grief and eventual euphoria can happen when tension is released in the body. All the effort used to maintain those inefficient and unconscious body/mind holding patterns are exhausting. Once released, that energy can be better spent creating a life with less pain and restriction. It is an honor to witness this phenomenon even as it is some times heart breaking to watch and know what all that tension in the body has robbed a person of over their life. Not everyone is ready or willing to use therapeutic body work like this, but those that are ready and willing, find relief from some persistent physical and mental conditions. The body is a fine teacher if you make friends with it, get acquainted with it, offer it the chance to soften, relax and let go. A strong, flexible, upright posture supports not only homeostasis but a more positive outlook on life. Some times the act of looking at the horizon instead of at the floor can create a fundamental shift in perspective that reverberates far and wide. There will be more on this topic in the chapter on Movement.

Again I must remind us all, this is not your garden variety quick fix, this is slow moments of self realization that accumulate over time. If an interest in what makes you tick begins to emerge, there is hope. If there is a realization about what helps you take a deeper breath, what allows ease of movement in body and mind, you may be on the path. If you can slow down and endure your own bodily sensations and thoughts without moving to suppress, hide or trivialize them, you have begun. If you can contemplate what helps you place meaning in and feel joy from the basic gifts of being alive as a human being, you can slowly begin to build fortitude and strength. You may be on your way to realizing you are a human being, full of potential and beauty and therefore full of inherent worth. It does not happen over night, in a week, a month or a year. It is an on going Restoration Project that requires the utmost patience and kindness as glimmers of self acceptance begin to be developed. Things get a little clearer and lighter relatively quick, even as The Project continues. We are not looking for perfection over night, we are looking for steady progress and a more realistic regard for our humanness and innate value and worth.

Movement Is Medicine

There is no concrete line between body and mind that says: *this is where the mind ends and the body begins.* The mind permeates the body and the body can exert a very strong influence over the health of the mind.

A body in motion will tend to stay in motion, a body at rest will tend to stay at rest unless some force of exertion is applied. Remember Sir Isaac Newton? His three Laws of Motion have been verified time and again and if you consider the motion processes in the body that maintain health due to strength, fluidity and movement it is no surprise that a strong, fluid and adaptable body will be a valuable part of creating a strong, fluid, adaptable mind. This fundamental pillar of health will serve you well into your senior years if you nurture and maintain proper care of yourself. Exercise! Stretching, strength building, and movement are medicine for the body/mind. Exercise can build stronger brain cognition, release held physical and mental tension, reduce inflammation and blood pressure, build strong bones, muscles and organs and release far more feel good neurotransmitters like serotonin and dopamine into the blood stream than any cigarette, can of soda or cookie ever has.[36]

Feel worthy of all that care and maintenance, know you deserve it, consider and contemplate little by little that you are a valuable and miraculous human being until you believe it. There is simply no possible way that you are a worthless piece of nothing. It took somewhere around nine months to make you (not to mention thousands of years for humans to evolve into what we are today), and regardless of the circumstances that brought you into this world, the fact that you are here against all odds even, makes you a survivor. It makes you a strong, worthy, beautiful human being worth every care and kindness even if you currently have a shell of lies about your worth covering over your human potential, your power and beauty are there waiting for you. Believe it—it's true.

---

36 American Physiological Society (2011, July 25). Exercise has numerous beneficial effects on brain health and cognition,

Chapter Highlights and Suggestions

Negative and self destructive thoughts effect not just the mind but the body as well. Getting hip to your thoughts can offer insight into your mental operating system and how self limiting thoughts may be subconsciously driving your behavior and your physical well-being.

- Dealing with the subconscious is a process—do not have unrealistic expectations there are no magic bullets.

- Begin to slow your mind down long enough to hear the subconscious thoughts that run through it all day long. Pay attention to your thoughts right now. Even for just a few minutes.

- Ask about a thought you may catch in your mindfulness experiment. Is it true? Is it kind? Is it helpful? Would you say it out loud in the presence of another person?

- If it would hurt a friendship to say it out loud, why would you say it to yourself, about yourself?

- The poison is the same whether you say a negative thought to yourself or out loud.

- Let negative thoughts go a million times until they lose their sting. Remember it is a process!

- Reframe, Reframe, Reframe! Check out the Reframe Revolution: www.designtoawaken.com/RR/Reframe_Revolution_Home.html

- The brain is "plastic" meaning new neural pathways can be created with your thoughts, this will in turn change your mental outlook and feed your body with uplifting information.

- **The next time you do or say something kind to someone, say and do those things for yourself as well.**

- **Consider therapeutic bodywork to help you gain insight into how your postural patterns inform your quality of life.**

- **Move your body daily, it will help release stagnant thoughts and keep you strong and fluid.**

- **Positive thoughts are restorative!**

Resiliency and Accepting What Is

"Success is stumbling from failure to failure with no loss of enthusiasm."

—Winston Churchill

Inner fortitude, adaptability and the capacity for a person to return to their original state after being disturbed is the hallmark of some of the greatest success stories of our time. From people like Nelson Mandela and Abraham Lincoln to Steve Jobs, and J. K. Rowling we can see examples of triumph after failure. Each of them suffered and lost many times before their resiliency paid off. In J. K. Rowling's June 2008 Commencement Address at the Annual Meeting of the Harvard Alumni Association she shares her thoughts on resiliency in a speech titled : *"The Fringe Benefits of Failure and the Importance of Imagination."* Rowlings shares many words of advice on moving forward through adversity, and one of my favorites from the speech was this:

"It is impossible to live without failing at something, unless you live so cautiously that you might as well not have lived at all—in which case, you fail by default."

RESILIENCY AND ACCEPTING WHAT IS

And this:

> *"Life is difficult, and complicated, and beyond anyone's total control, and the humility to know that will enable you to survive its vicissitudes."*

I think it is better to have tried and failed than to never have tried at all, don't you? At some point the trying could very well lead to something very important, even if it doesn't look like what you thought it would look like and most especially if you had to struggle to achieve it.

Many people have described this concept of building strength through trial and error, from Buddhist re-framing and Byron Katie's "The Work" to a host of bloggers, writers and life coaches who recommend we accept *what is* instead of the self torture we endure when we convince ourselves things should be other than they are. Cultivating an attitude of responsiveness and adaptability to life circumstances is good for our central nervous system, no matter how you describe or define it.

Resiliency is like a muscle that grows strong when exercised. In time it can become a choice. The kind of choice that comes along with the burden of being creatures endowed with Free Will. It is clear that we can choose how we frame things, how we place meaning upon things and this has a huge bearing on how content and at ease we feel in the world. Every situation we are faced with has an inherent multiplicity within it. We can choose to see the situation as an opportunity, with an unknowable future out come that we perhaps can't see yet, or we can see it as the foreboding of a most terrible disaster and allow it to plunge us into building a riveting and compelling case for bad luck and giving up. Often times these things that may be seen as a terrible stroke of bad luck lead us to opportunities we may never have been exposed to other wise.

For example, a client of mine found herself laid-off from a high paying corporate job. This job was draining but gave her a sense of security, despite the fact that she was laid off and flung into losing the safety net she came to trust would always be there. She had developed skills and many contacts through this job, and began to look for the opportunities that laid buried within the lay off. As she worked with new ideas, momentum started to build. In time, she began to see the workings of a consulting business idea. She reached out and did the ground work that in time grew to be a successful business of her own. This job paid more and allowed her to create her own schedule. For the first time in her life she began to take real vacations and her stress level started to come down. She realized how tired she had become from the demands of the corporate world, how it had slowly begun to erode her happiness and state of mind. With the new found space she created in her life she began to contemplate starting a family due to having more time, and resources. In under two years her entire life blossomed and she began to recapture her authentic self. She created this opportunity from the inner strength she did not know she had, that may have remained dormant had the "misfortune" of being laid off not presented itself. She also learned from this process that taking risks is something she can do now. She developed a trust in herself and the world around her and developed potential she did not know she had. Watching this process of empowerment unfold not only enriched her life, but the lives of those around her, including mine. As I watched this scenario unfold, I asked if it would be okay to share her experience with other clients who come in with similar stories. With a smile she agreed, happy to consider that her experience could help others. Burn out, disenchantment, mental and physical deterioration and unmanageable stress levels are a familiar life-sketch of the majority of folks us body workers treat on a daily basis. Her story has lived on every time I or anyone else relates it to others. I cannot really say how many people it has touched. Maybe by just planting one seed for someone who wishes they could shift their current situation, her courage has given the spark of hope to others.

We often have to hear something hundreds of times before we act, we often live in great misery before we either create change or change is created for us despite our enormous capacity to endure. When one person breaks free, the potential is there for that one act to support another in their efforts. When one of us rises, it paves the way for others. I see this shift happening as people grow less and less enamored of the corporate model. That model has changed, it is no longer a fair distribution of company wealth, it is no longer a road to comfortable retirement to stay in one job for the better part of one's life all while keeping an eye on the company matched pension. People have lost trust and faith for good reason and something new is beginning to emerge. Every time someone chooses to leave that tattered corporate fairy-tale it hauls the rest of us up into the bright and hopeful light of reality and helps us to see that there is another way to live that is less soul crushing. By soul crushing I mean not only for each person as an individual but also for the planet. Abandoning the greedy, destructive corporate model is not just good for us humans, but it is critical for the survival of life on this planet.

> *"If I were asked to give what I consider the single most useful bit of advice for all humanity, it would be this: Expect trouble as an inevitable part of life, and when it comes, hold your head high. Look it squarely in the eye, and say, 'I am bigger than you. You cannot defeat me'."*
>
> —Ann Landers

The Hero's Journey

Since we are bringing up matters of evolving lives, systems and ideas I'll take this another step and add that resiliency, could even include returning to your original state having gained something of great value from the experience of de-stabilization or disturbance. You do not return from the experience the same as you were, but stronger. Perhaps you may even gain insight, wisdom and confidence from the experience. Which feeds right into the concept of The Hero's Journey, a term coined by Joseph Campbell who was known for his work in comparative mythology and religion. In the making of any hero, we see an ordinary person in their ordinary world, but then from out of nowhere a call to enter an unknown world of strange powers and unordinary happenings is offered or some times thrust upon them. The person who accepts the call to enter this strange world must face challenges, tasks and trials, at times alone but often at the perfect moment, help arrives. If the hero survives, he or she may achieve attributes, or gifts that perhaps even possess a supernatural quality to them. The hero must then decide whether to return to the ordinary world with this new found strength and power. If the hero does decide to return, he or she often faces challenges on the return journey, but upon returning successfully, the gifts they've acquired may be used to improve the world.

Greek and Egyptian mythology are full of fine examples of the Hero's Journey as are most major religions from Christianity to Buddhism. Many of our most beloved and popular books and movies are based upon a hero character facing great challenges and over coming fear, hardship, loneliness and even death, to return in triumph as a changed and stronger person.

> *"Certainty of death...small chance of success...what are we waiting for?"*
>
> *Gimli, son of Gloin before the battle of Helms Deep in Rohan.*
> *—The Lord of the Rings, movie screen play*
> *by Peter Jackson and Philippa Boyens*

My favorite tales of the Hero's Journey for decades have been the books of Professor J. R. R Tolkien in his epic Silmarillion, Hobbit, and Lord of the Rings stories. The Hobbit legacy begins when one Bilbo

RESILIENCY AND ACCEPTING WHAT IS

Baggins, a well respected Hobbit of The Shire, is visited by Gandalf the Gray, a great wizard. Gandalf has felt in his heart that this humble and unassuming Hobbit would be the perfect addition to the thirteen dwarf companions looking to reclaim their ancestral home far away in Erebor, from the terror of the dragon Smaug. "Why me?" asks Bilbo, "I am just a humble Hobbit, with no possible skills for such a quest, surely you must have the wrong person!" He refuses at first, with fear and insecurity claiming him. All the elements of The Hero's Journey are met by Bilbo in his long journey to the mountain and back again: he is happily living in the ordinary, he receives the call to adventure, he meets mentors along the way, he is tested many times, he finds allies, makes it through the supreme ordeal, finds the elixir, and experiences a certain kind of resurrection and ultimate return to ordinary life carrying the reward. It all begins when the undeniable call to adventure takes over and Bilbo rushes out the door after the dwarves for the adventure of a life time. He faces everything from trolls, goblins, cold and hunger, to insecurity and close brushes with death. Yet in the end, he proves not only to himself but the entire company that he is an irreplaceable and valued member of the group. What we see in the end is a Bilbo Baggins who has developed self confidence, great strength, compassion and wisdom. In fact the unlooked for help in the form of a ring which makes the bearer invisible proves to be a great boon for Mister Baggins. A super power if you will, is bestowed upon him through the ring. It is not until much later in the tales that we learn this ring is the One Ring, it is evil in fact and must be destroyed. Bilbo passes his penchant for adventure to his young nephew Frodo, through his legendary stories of elves, dragons and great mountain lands far away. We have the great pleasure of watching yet another hero being reluctantly pulled out of The Shire with Frodo finishing what his uncle started in *The Lord of the Rings*.

Tolkien's books have gained slow but steady popularity over the years and were catapulted into total cultural acceptance after Peter Jackson produced his wonderful interpretations of the books as movies. The

Lord of the Rings grossed almost ten million per movie. [37] The movies became one of the biggest box office smash hits of all time, winning seventeen Oscar Awards. The Lord of the Rings became a household name beloved by millions. The numbers for The Hobbit movies are not yet fully known at the writing of this book but I'm sure they will equally demonstrate that the concept of the Hero's Journey is one of great interest to large numbers of people. These epic stories of triumph over hardship capture the human imagination on a primal archetypal level for a reason. We all want to believe that hero is within us. We admire and perhaps secretly wish to be that hero. Our heroes are held in high regard and we want them to succeed, we live through them from the safety of the movie theater, or pages of books perhaps with a quiet yearning for an adventure of our own.

I believe we all possess these noble and honorable gifts, hidden deep, buried under the lies we've been told about not being good enough. We may feel that we do not have access to the greatness required to live a life of unpredictable challenges, and perhaps at first that is true. Yet we see time and again the strength that is required appears, or is built along the way. Clearly the journey itself creates and magnifies our inherent but untapped potential. We may not have possessed such power at the beginning of the journey, but we most surely possess it in the end. It is cultivated out of adversity and without being presented with these things that strain the edges of our capabilities we may never know what we are really made of.

If we can reframe our greatest tests as yet another step on the hero's journey we may be able to greet the challenges with hope, and gather our strength with faith in ourselves to see it through. At the heart of resiliency is this very concept. If we can grow to see that the universe is always conspiring to help us evolve into our greatest selves we may begin to look at life as a great adventure. It may appear over whelming

---

37 "Movie Franchises". *The Numbers*. Nash Information Services. Retrieved September 24, 2011.

at first to leave that unfulfilling job, go back to school in our forties, move to a new country, write that book, or take that dream road trip across the country. We may find that if we take the leap, the help we need to complete the task will appear just at the perfect moment. We may not at first be able to see how it will all work out but that is part of what builds the strength and wisdom that becomes the super power in the end. To enter an unknown experience with no guarantee of success is a necessary component in building strength. The beginning may not look like what we think it should look like, perhaps no wizards will appear and we may not come across any magic rings but these are metaphors and encouragements to keep in mind to stand strong and resilient in the face of our fears.

The Hero's Journey is one we all may have to take in our lives and with any luck at all we answer the call of adventure and embark upon perhaps the most challenging but rewarding tale of our lives. In fact I think the entirety of one's life could be considered a Hero's Journey as this pilgrimage could most certainly take a lifetime to complete. The first step Joseph Campbell defines in the journey is "The Call to Adventure." Some answer the call to adventure, others do not but at times when the call happens, circumstances may not allow a refusal. Perhaps those "unlucky" people are luckiest of all.

Chapter Highlights and Suggestions

Begin to increase your inner fortitude by seeing challenges as opportunities that in time, will leave you stronger and wiser.

- Take heart in the stories of your own heroes who failed before they could succeed.

- When "misfortune" happens look for what is positive within in. Make *it* work for *you*.

- Trust that quiet voice inside that is yearning to grow or have an adventure.

- Test the edges of your abilities frequently, when you find freedom and strength you may inspire others who yearn to grow.

- Even if you can't see the whole picture, take the first steps and look for the help that may appear along the way. Plan what you can but leave room for the fates to do their work!

- Your situation may not look like what you think it should look like, look again! Reframe!

- Growth is rarely comfortable, it's in the struggle that strength is built.

- Take in uplifting stories of adventure for inspiration. Read books or watch movies about the topic .

- If the Call to Adventure happens, answer it with even a shaky and tentative *yes*.

- Surround yourself with adventurous people, watch them carefully and learn.

- Reach out for help through coaching, therapy and positive, supportive friends.

Here's a great resource: The Reframe Revolution

www.designtoawaken.com/RR/Reframe_Revolution_Coaching.html

The Art of Living

"When the artist is alive in any person, what ever his/her kind of work may be, he/she becomes an inventive, searching, daring, self-expressing creature. He/she disturbs, upsets, enlightens and opens ways for a better understanding"

—Robert Henri

What does it mean to create a work of art out of life? What might it look like? What might it feel like? Like most concepts here, there is no singular right way, and that is the beauty of it. There is no starting point and no ending point. It starts the moment you choose it and ends, perhaps never. To create a work of art of one's life is a living concept that will constantly evolve as you move through your days. The artful life is resilient, and adaptable, and sees adventure and beauty in the mundane. Creating an artful life takes concentration and thoughtfulness and of course it takes time. Allowing space and time in life is a conscious choice. It is the choice to let some things go in order to allow deeper things to emerge and many of us may find that a challenge and a sacrifice. Can you let those emails sit for a short time in favor of a walk outside? I would propose to you that it is a worthy endeavor that will deliver some portion of a remedy for so many of us craving more space with our own thoughts. Our innate humanness yearns for meaning, connection and beauty and this requires time and space for the meaning of life to settle within and express itself outward.

Does this imply that some part of the meaning of life is to recognize and amplify beauty? I would encourage you to think about it, see what it means to you to not only recognize beauty but to create it in your life. It doesn't have to be a painting, or a symphony to be a beautiful feeling or expression of artful living. The way you smile at a stranger could be an artful act. Placing a vase of flowers on the table or sending a hand written note to a friend to let them know you are thinking of them could be an expression of an artful life. A colorful, juicy bowl of fruit in the morning that gently nourishes your senses could be considered an artful first meal of the day.

Running through life breathless and hurried is the opposite of art because rushing kills art. The artistic endeavor is a certain vision, feeling or insight with meaning breathed into it, that the world may have missed if not for the artist calling our attention to it in some way that touched or moved us. Art has the power to remind us of some long forgotten memory, passion, joy, or sorrow. That may be why in some ways we exalt the artist, and have great respect and ardor for the person who can make us feel something so human, so authentic and raw.

I haven't known a single person who has not had the experience of being moved by some form of art. It could be a song, a movie, a painting, a sculpture, a book, a poem, or a piece of gorgeous clothing. What ever medium it lives through, art has the power to keep us human and inspire us. It could even take the form of being inspired and uplifted by a person who lives a life full of kindness and generosity.

It is the human condition to respond to art and I think there is some part of an artist living, some times buried, within us all. What if more days in the week are spent living our very lives as if they are beautiful human works of art? What if we begin to see the beauty in a patch of wild flowers somehow thriving on a busy highway, or the birds nest perched on a rusty old road sign, or the miraculous way life pushes its way through the cement as grass reaches its way up through the pavement. There are moments in every day that may begin to appear more vibrant than you've noticed before, that is the essence of living the artful life. Whether you find a way to outwardly express how life touches you or not is your business alone. Some of us are compelled to find a way to express it, but for some it may simply be a personal experience that makes life more colorful and interesting.

Beauty and art are every where if you see with artful eyes. For example, a child giggling in line at the grocery store could bring an internal giggle to the observer bringing a moment of child-like joy to the day. Noticing two friends talking at the coffee shop clearly enjoying each others' company could bring a fond memory of your own friendships. The driver before you who waves you into a long line of traffic with a smile, or even better, you allow someone into your line of traffic with a smile. Oh how engaging it is to create an artful moment of grace and kindness any time you choose to. Look for the opportunities, they are every where.

Nourishment for the Senses

The Art of Living is a sensory experience, it requires paying special attention to sights, smells, sounds, tastes and feelings and then awarding them the value they deserve. Many people have built barriers around their sensory system, actively dulling their responses to all that they take in. Over time the world becomes dull and meaningless like a plane of glass covered in grime. All the while they are holding a bottle of glass cleaner and a cloth in their hands that they have forgotten they can use. Reawakening the senses requires some effort and action. Can you take a daily walk in the woods and notice, really *see, smell, hear and feel* the forest, the beach or a pretty neighborhood in your town. Lay on the grass and look up at the morning or evening sky, the clouds and the stars truly are miraculous if you learn to see them that way. Notice the little details, it is there that you find the art. Notice how the fading light of day casts that haunting glow over the landscape. Notice the tilt of a head as someone listens to a song, a friend talking about some current event, the sparkle in their eye, the expression on their face, what put it there? Feel it, give it meaning, honor and acknowledge the range of human expression and feeling. A trip to the florist or the park or city gardens, reading a passage in an inspirational book, talking with a friend, listening to music, or taking a few moments to write some lines in your journal can all begin to stir and awaken the artist within. Can you choose to take your lunch outside for a picnic instead of eating at your desk? Pretend as if you have a date with The Muse. If you show up, with open eyes, ears and heart, she really wants to appear although she cannot be rushed. So have patience.

It doesn't require affluence or power to interact with any of the aforementioned things. It only requires an inquisitive and open attitude and of course that ever elusive "time." You may notice many of the suggestions here come straight out of the natural world around us. Another benefit of seeing, feeling, hearing, smelling and tasting the beauty that abounds in nature is once you have connected with it, you will no longer be able to tolerate the destruction of it. If the world contained within it, more people who are nourished and inspired by earthly splendor, the harder it would be to desecrate it.

Try it for a week and see how you feel after the week is over. More calm and settled inside, more content perhaps? If you observe even a little feeling of change inside after the week, try a second week. Take a break and go back to your skim-the-surface-style of living and see how it feels. Become a scientist, do your experiment, make your observations and decide for yourself if seeding this into your life adds value. Maybe you decide you will have one week per month where you allow your inner artist to get some exercise and see if over time, it naturally begins to become two weeks or more. Notice what begins to happen throughout your days of artful living.

> "May morning be astir with the harvest of night;
> Your mind quickening to the Eros of a new question,
> Your eyes seduced by some unintended glimpse
> That cut right through the surface to a source."
>
> —*John O'Donahue*

Chapter Highlights and Suggestions

Take a moment to define for yourself what it means to embrace The Art of Living. Write it down, refer to it often, add to it as new ideas emerge. A few keys words/phrases to get you started:

- Seeing beauty in the mundane.

- Relying on your senses to help you feel the world more acutely, (stop to smell, look, feel, see, hear and appreciate the flowers, birds, bees, clouds, stars, people and landscape around you!)

- Allow yourself to place meaning upon what you find beautiful.

Creating time and space in your day for developing Artful Living Habits

- Can those emails wait a little before you respond?

- Favor a walk/picnic outside instead of eating lunch at your desk.

- Court The Muse and Be Patient! She needs to know you are serious about the relationship!

- Notice the details; the way the light hits just so, the tilt of a head, one petal missing from a flower, a mama bird feeding her baby.

- Utilize time when kids are in school to wander, be alert to, and notice the details you encounter, record them or just feel them and allow yourself to be nourished and restored.

- Do not underestimate the power of tuning into the earth, the healing and inspiration of the earth never ceases.

- See the chapter called Touch the Earth for more.

Become a Scientist

- Make your observations.

- Decide if they add value.

- Try living slower and deeper for a day/week then go back to the hurried skim-the-surface-living and see if you can go back and forth to tease out your preferences.

Take your Artful Living habits out for a spin perhaps one day or one week per month and see if gradually over time you naturally begin to prefer the depth of living a more conscious Artful Life.

Meditation and Stillness

"Work is not always required. There is such a thing as sacred idleness."

—*George MacDonald*

What would our Restoration Project be without the vitally important practice of meditation? We've saved the best for last as they say. Meditation; the art and practice of training the central nervous system to be calm, the scientifically proven method of developing compassion, concentration, and patience. The practice of contemplation and stillness has been deeply embedded into most cultures, religions and spiritual traditions since the beginning of recorded history. So what is it about the staying power of going within, that has followed human cultures through so many centuries when many other things have come and gone over time? Universal truths tend to have that staying power. They may come in and out of favor somewhat but there has not been a time in history where the practice of inner reflection has disappeared from the face of the earth. There have been devoted lineages and traditions studying, practicing and reaping the benefits of meditation continuously for centuries.

There are a variety of ways to approach the practice, there is not a right way or a wrong way, only the way that fits the constitution, personality, and preference of the person meditating at any given time in their life. So let us begin by answering the question of: why meditate? For many people it may seem a fruitless waste of time when there is so much that needs doing. We are gradually training our minds to multitask and it may seem like all that multitasking is creating more productive and effective people so really, there is no time to meditate, right? How can we just sit there, when there are so many things we cannot get to even if we work continuously through the day, right?

Well lets take a look, lets see if it is true that a multitasking mind is more effective than a mind that takes regular productive quiet time and is able to focus upon one thing at a time and see it through to a conclusion.

Multitasking by definition is the act of doing several activities simultaneously, although in reality it is more accurate to say it is switching back and forth between tasks and doing several things in rapid succession. So you may be working away at your lap top with your phone at the ready to instantly fire back at any incoming texts or phone calls that may come in. At the same time you may be toggling back and forth between computer screens perhaps checking email, Facebook and Twitter while researching information at work etc. Your brain is skimming the surface of four or five tasks at once and lets imagine then that someone comes into your office to ask a question. Can you put yourself there right now? How does it feel when another person comes in and disturbs this chaotic and fast moving machine you've created there at your desk? Are you annoyed? Irritated? Do you know somewhere inside that any external influence has the power to topple that whole juggling act apart because you barely know what you are doing yourself? Do you leave work at the end of the day feeling like very little got done, adding to your anxiety and stress about finishing tasks both at work and in your personal life? Take heart because you are not alone. A culture of rapid fire information sharing has got many heads spinning. All this fast moving information can create an inner sense of urgency and tension that seeps into every day existence with no "off" switch in sight. It happens so gradually that it may even be difficult to know what has happened to your sense of ease, except that under all your exhaustion, you know you are hosting chaos.

There are things you can do to harness your concentration and effectiveness even in this chaotic world. At one time you may have been very good at focusing on a task for long periods of time. In childhood it comes naturally, kids can immerse for hours if they find interest in something. With a little dedication you can recapture a sense of calm that will leave you feeling satisfied and content with your daily activities. Research shows time and again that the human brain was not designed for task switching, as much as it was for integrative focus. Meaning, we can focus on a few related things at once quite well, but switching back and forth between mediums and subject matter, not so well.

Say for example, you are writing a paper on the gypsy moth caterpillar and you have several sources open; photos of the gypsy moth, an audio file and other basic written information about their habitat and life cycle. The sources may be mixed media but all are about the same topic, you can read a bit, then at the completion of a chapter, have a look at some visual aids which is a different kind of information, all adding to what you just read. The brain can work with this, deepening your understanding on the subject matter. Yet if you are doing three or four totally unrelated things at once, details get missed, retention is low, and comprehension suffers. The human brain was not designed well for multitasking evolutionarily speaking. We may be pressing the envelope and perhaps future generations will come in with brains wired for skimming the surface. Right now however, task switching produces anxiety due to incomplete comprehension of subject matter and injecting chaos into our lives. It also has detrimental side effects on areas of human personality. Culture will adapt to this level of shallow comprehension, in fact I see signs of that already happening. Some have coined the phrase, *"The Dumming Down of America."* I don't like that phrase, do you?

The trend of having several screens with different subject matter flashing and buzzing away catches our attention pulling us into ever increasing and endless scrolling, researching and communication, but it has also brought a whole new dimension of distraction to the fore front, making us far less productive in the long run. Add texting and scrolling while driving, or checking out at the market, or meeting a friend for coffee, or playing with your kids, and you begin to miss out on being in your real life. This has hit such proportions as to be the topic of a variety of research studies, and the outcomes are disturbing to say the least.

We met Clifford Nass back in our Going Unplugged chapter, and we will meet him again here. Clifford Nass was a professor in the Communications department at Stanford, with additional positions in Computer Science, Education, Law, and Sociology. He was also affiliated with the programs in Technology, and Society and Cognitive Science. In 2009 Nass conducted studies comparing both heavy and light media users with a research method called a trait media multitasking index.[38] These two groups were compared along the established cognitive control study guidelines. The results showed clearly that those who engaged in heavy media task switching are less able to filter out non-relevant information and they performed worse on task switching tests compared to their light media multitasking counterparts. In another study by David Sanbonmatsu and his research team from the Department of Psychology at the University of Utah, a group of undergrads where asked to memorize a sequence of letters interspersed with simple math equations.[39] The students were also evaluated to de-

---

38 Cognitive Control in Media Multitaskers, Eyal Ophir, Clifford Nass,b,1 and Anthony D. Wagnerc v.106(37); Sep 15, 2009PMC2747164
39 Sanbonmatsu, D. M., Strayer, D. L., Medeiros-Ward, N., and Watson, J. M. (2013).

termine their habits of multitasking and media device usage. Those who performed poorly on the test showing weak memory and cognition were the most frequent multitaskers, yet this group also held the belief that they had a greater degree of productivity even though the opposite was actually proven to be true. Those same people were also more likely to drive while texting and scored high for impulsive and sensation-seeking behavior. Co-author of the Utah study David Strayer reported that; "The people who multitask the most tend to be impulsive, sensation-seeking, overconfident of their multitasking abilities, and tend to be less capable of multitasking."

It is also not clear just what kind of damage to cognitive ability occurs through long term multitasking. There is enough information out there now to prove that our multitasking habits are not making us more productive, so why wait to begin introducing time into every day to practice some simple exercises to neutralize the never ending stream of chaos that has engulfed and taken over our lives?

In another study assistant professor at Ohio State University Zheng Wang had college students record all of their media use and other activities for twenty-eight days, including why they used various media sources and what they got out of it. [40] The findings showed that multitasking often gave the students an emotional boost, even while it hurt cognitive functions, such as studying. Let us not mistake the feel good sensation of constant media distraction with productivity.

There is mounting evidence that multiple distractions invading our minds makes us less focused, less accurate, and less productive. Constant mental busyness increases our stress response and creates agitation and impatience as well. So can we agree that although it may feel good

---

Multi-tasking ability, perceived multi-tasking ability, impulsivity, and sensation seeking. PLoS ONE, 8(1), e54402. doi:10.1371/journal.pone.0054402

40 Wang, Zheng, and John M. Tchernev. 2012. "The 'Myth' of Media Multitasking: Reciprocal Dynamics of Media Multitasking, Personal Needs, and Gratifications." Journal of Communication 62 (3): 493-513. doi:10.1111/j.1460-2466.2012.01641.x.

and fill some other kind of void inside, multitasking is most certainly not the fast track to productivity that we think it is? What is the alternative? How can we slowly train ourselves to focus on one thing at a time, if not at least several related things at once? Or at the very least create time in every day for the mind to rest so when we return to work, we do so refreshed and more able to concentrate. There is nothing glamorous about allowing so much busyness in our lives that we are tense, spaced out, unfocused and just plain old chaotic. Multitasking is wearing away our nerves little by little exhausting us from deep inside, it needs to change and we are the only ones who can do that for ourselves. There is plenty of help around now, making it easier to change habits but we have to make the choice to seek it out and practice it a little bit every day until it becomes a normal part of life.

> *"The mind is a superb instrument if used rightly. Used wrongly, however, it becomes very destructive. To put it more accurately, it is not so much that you use your mind wrongly—you usually don't use it at all. It uses you. This is the disease. You believe that you are your mind. This is the delusion. The instrument has taken you over."*
>
> —Eckhart Tolle

Meditation

Meditation is one way to expand the capacity of your brain to concentrate as well as having a calming effect upon the central nervous system. A nervous system that has become trained to stay on high alert can create a variety of nervous disorders, everything from migraines, muscle pain, insomnia, panic attacks, high blood pressure, teeth clenching, anger, anxiety and depression—to name only a few. The word "stress" has become a catch-all phrase for the cause of many life style related illnesses and in some ways the word has lost some meaning, even though we know ongoing stress is destructive to health and well being. Many people go to the doctor about high levels of stress and come away with a prescription to help increase serotonin in the brain as a way to ease the effects of stress. Even when less than half of the people given those medications actually respond well. Some times it is not a serotonin problem at all. Or people take an anti anxiety pill, once called tranquilizers, and endure the side effects in the hopes of easing their habit of not being able to relax. Anti anxiety drugs are not a cure but often times they are used as if they were, despite the side effects which range from memory loss, nausea and depression to mental lethargy confusion and impaired thinking. After we have altered our chemistry with expensive drugs and grown tired of the side effects perhaps then we will see there are long term solutions that come with no side effects, and other side benefits that begin to spill into many other areas of our lives. I dare say, engaging in relaxation practices can be a cure for the over stimulated nervous system, if only we would give it a chance and understand that nature heals slowly, but heal She does. Drugs are an illusory "quick fix" offering only short term benefits riddled with diminishing returns, while relaxation practices have a compounding benefit that begin to pay dividends that have shown themselves to be the best investment of time that any of us could make to enhance our quality of life and the lives of those around us. Like any other activity it takes practice to get good at it, especially if you have spent many years locked in hyper vigilance.

The Power of Relaxation

In a most basic way, relaxation can happen any time and any where you choose that is appropriate. Really, it can, and it is free! You own it! No one can take it from you. Slowly training your central nervous system to relax is the beginning of learning to meditate. Relaxation is the key to internal happiness and health—I am utterly convinced of this. It seems to me that many of us are not even sure what it fees like to be relaxed any more. Very often that surrendered, peaceful state of being, left the scene somewhere just before puberty and has not been felt since. Have you been in a deep state of relaxation lately? Do you remember what it feels like to be free of tension in your muscles, and possess a mind that is not bent on being worried, over stimulated, or impatient? Have you slept well and awakened refreshed on a regular basis? Can you take a full deep breath and not be met with restriction in your rib cage or belly? Is the back of your neck supple and soft, or hard and tense? Do you suffer from pain and stiffness in your neck, jaw or shoulders? All of these areas are the frontline of symptoms when your central nervous system has become locked in "fight or flight" mode, or locked in a chronic stress response over too much time. The neck, jaw, shoulders, and belly take a personal interest in the state of your central nervous system. If you are feeling chronic pain and tension in these areas learning how to relax could have a dramatic impact and go a long way in easing the root cause of the manifestation of chronic tension in your body/mind.

Basic relaxation is something you can practice throughout your day. Notice if you are clenching your teeth, tensing your shoulders or neck and consciously take a breath in and soften those hard places. At your desk, in the car, before bed, and upon rising are all fine times to practice. Of course you can also set aside a specific time, create a special place, and sink in deeper for longer periods of time once the feeling of relaxation becomes comfortable. There are workshops on meditation, books, digital guided meditations, retreats and group practice all designed to support you in your efforts. Start small and build up. Done with even a little consistency the benefits of relaxation that lead into meditation can be felt early on in your practice. It is called practice because it is an ongoing activity that accumulates over time to restore the mind and body. In time your body and mind will overflow with inner peace and calmness.

Meditation has been shown to regulate heart beat, deepen the breath, clear the mind and relax the muscles, along with a host of beneficial physiological changes in the brain. Richard Davidson Professor of Psychology and Psychiatry at the University of Wisconsin-Madison has conducted several research projects both with John Kabbat Zinn and The Dalai Lama to discover exactly what happens in the brains of experienced meditators.[41] [42]What was discovered during some of these research experiments at the home of the Dalai Lama in India, has been published and republished over the years and has nurtured a great interest on the part of The Dalai Lama. Joining meditation and neuroscience together for the benefit of humanity is an area of great interest to The Dalai Lama that he is obviously excited about sharing.

What is so uplifting about the Dalai Lama's invitations to study his brain and the brains of other monks in his company makes perfect sense. If you want to learn about how to generate ease, happiness and health, study the brains of people who have achieved it. Instead of focusing on pathology, focus on recreating the brain health found in a population of people who have been shown to have an enormous amount of compassion, well being and happiness. Just like Edward Bach did with his flower essences, health can be created by amplifying the virtuous qualities and leaving pathology to resolve in the light of that virtue. The Dalai Lama is essentially saying the same thing that Edward Bach was saying. If you have never been in the presence of The Dalai Lama I highly recommend it. He travels quite a bit giving lectures that are wonderfully uplifting events. I can only describe being in his presence as healing. His effervescence spills over into the room where people are prone to smiling, joking, laughing, and generally getting over themselves in a most delightful way. Do I want more of that? You bet I do! Clearly this kind of happiness is not hinged upon circum-

---

41 Davidson, R. J.; Kabat-Zinn, J.; Schumacher, J.; Rosenkranz, M.; Muller, D.; Santorelli, S.; Urbanowski, F.; Harrington, A.; Bonus, K.; Sheridan, J. F. (2003). "Alterations in Brain and Immune Function Produced by Mindfulness Meditation". *Psychosomatic Medicine* 65 (4): 564–570. doi:10.1097/01.PSY.0000077505.67574.E3. PMID 12883106. edit

42 Davidson, Richard J.; Harrington, Anne, eds. (December 6, 2001). Visions of Compassion: Western Scientists and Tibetan Buddhists Examine Human Nature. New York: Oxford University Press. p. 288. 978-0-19-513043-0.

stance, when we see what the Dalai Lama has experienced in his life. From great loss of his culture and the genocide of his people, to exile from his homelands, he has maintained his humanity and continues to be a positive force of healing for the world.

Using functional MRI technology, a variety of studies have been conducted with the Dalai Lama and his company of monks that show consistent meditation can promote a variety of emotional states like compassion, empathy, kindness and attention. Developing these traits has the ability to keep the body and mind healthy and highly functioning without the use of drugs or other substances. In another study with a monk that has been named Lama Oser researchers watched his brain through the *f* MRI machine enter an "open state." This to me is the among the highest aspirations for meditation being used as a tool for developing a high level of consciousness and restoration. The "open state" is a thought-free wakefulness where the mind, as Oser described it, "is open, vast and aware, with no intentional mental activity. The mind is not focused on anything, yet totally present—not in a focused way, just very open and undistracted. Thoughts may start to arise weakly, but they don't chain into longer thoughts—they just fade away."

The ultimate act of the Human Restoration Project is to reach an open/aware state as often as we can. This open state corresponds to slower brain waves which are associated with increased learning and memory. The open state also offers reduction in stress and the ability of the central nervous system to be tuned up, restored and repaired. It leaves us feeling released from the burdens of worry and agitation and in the absence of worry, what would we be? We'd be healthy, and happy. Just as stress cascades throughout the body via the vagus nerve, so does this "open state" cascade through the body sending messages of relaxation, peacefulness and contentment. We cannot get that feeling from a pill without serious detrimental side effects and I am beginning to understand that the act of having to engage in action is part of the medicine.

The easy come, easy go philosophy teaches us nothing. It builds no inner fortitude and no human power is cultivated when we are a passive recipient of some fleeting thing that comes out of a substance from an outside source. However, when we build something through deliberate action that comes from within, we amplify our human power and the healing switches get turned on from a potent place of pure health. Humans have potential that is laying dormant under a story we've all been told about doctors and medicine saving us from harm. Doctors and medicine can help of course, but they are about a third of the pie. The rest must come from within us.

Lets Do Another Experiment!

This basic recipe for a beginning meditation exercise can get you started, and if you find these suggestions helpful I encourage you to do some of your own research as there are many programs and supportive materials out there to keep you interested, growing and learning about how the Relaxation Response can contribute to, and enhance your life.

A Few Tips and Sample Meditation Exercises

To begin, sit up so that you can feel the boney protrusions at the base of your pelvis (the sitting bones or 'ischial tuberosities' for you anatomy geeks out there). You can sit in a chair with a back to support your spine, you can sit against a wall on the floor or sit under a tree or in your garden. There are meditation cushions and benches galore out there but you don't necessarily need one. A cushion, chair, couch or wall will do just fine. Make it a place with some level of privacy so you are not concerned with the possibility of being interrupted. Turn your phone all the way off and be some where that you cannot even see it or your lap top or iPad etc.

- Allow the eyes to close

- Soften the eye lids and relax the eyes.

- Allow space in the jaw so the top and bottom teeth are not touching.

- Bring the tongue to rest in the lower palate and note if it likes to adhere to the upper palate which stimulates brain activity. Just to keep your attention on your tongue can occupy your attention for quite some time! Aren't we fascinating us humans?

- Let the shoulders drop away from the ears, let gravity have them, feel your limbs getting heavy.

- Begin to place your attention on your breathing.

- Notice the inhale.

- Notice the exhale.

- Count the breath if your mind is chattering.

- No matter what just keep noticing the inhale and the exhale and the inner landscape of your body—that is your only job.

- Start with sitting like this for three minutes.

- Increase your time one minute at a time.

Start small and build. Start with three to five minutes and add a minute every few days. You may find you are naturally able to sit longer in a short period of time. This is one of countless methods and the end of this chapter has a list of books and programs to support you in your efforts. Do your own research in your area for classes, workshops and retreats. Being part of a meditation group is a wonderful and supportive way to maintain a consistent meditation habit. If you have a small alarm clock with a gentle alarm, set it for your three minutes so you don't have to concern yourself with the time. There are meditation timers and apps of course. Calm.com is a wonderful resource for meditation support with a timer, options for soothing music, and several different guided meditations you can try. You can download the app to your phone or to your lap top, although it might be nice to get into the habit of meditating away from the stimulating effects of the computer and phone. In a quiet electronically sparse room, or out in nature can be ideal environments for meditation. Also consider that many towns and cities have Buddhist and Zen meditation centers with rooms designed just for meditation.

Another easy beginner meditation is to repeat a word to yourself as you sit, to help you maintain focus. The word *peace* is a good one, or *relax*, *bliss*, or even just the word *stay*. If you notice your mind is wandering uttering the word *stay* to yourself can be a gentle way to train your body and mind to be still. If your body gets uncomfortable, you are not alone. Sitting still can bring up a variety of sensations not only in the mind but in the body. If your back begins to get stiff, know that this can happen and perhaps consider doing a little stretching before you sit. If discomfort arises allow yourself five breaths to simply be with the sensation and then in a mindful manner, slowly readjust your position or move into a walking meditation. Mindfully taking one step at a time, feeling the sensation of each part of your foot as it contacts the ground then again as it lifts off the ground. The idea is to remain focused and calm while walking which can be a wonderful way to begin seeding this more mindful disposition into more activities in your day.

Movement and Stillness—a Perfect Partnership

Meditation and physical exercise go hand in hand as do all of the other life affirming lifestyle choices included through the pages of this book. As you add more and more of those supportive activities to your life you will come to find they foster, support and build upon each other. They feed back and forth to strengthen and restore you. Less sugar and more real food has a calming effect on the brain as does exercise and stretching so as you move more and eat better it will become easier and easier to rest in meditative stillness. In time all your healthy habits will become normal and liberating. Yoga is a wonderful companion to meditation and the practice was developed as a way to prepare the body/mind for sitting in stillness for longer periods of time. Although when yoga hit the shores of North America, it became more about physical exercise, its origins in ancient India tell a more varied story. The Eight Limbs of the yogic system include far more than physical exercise. Using the breath and inner stillness to bring the mind into clarity and higher state of consciousness was considered among the most precious gifts of a regular yoga practice. Above all, the practice of sitting quietly and communing with your inner landscape serves to reunite you with the more subtle and omnipresent powers of your humanness. The breath and the mind are evolutionary change agents. When the potent forces of the mind and the breath are strengthened through regular yoga and meditation practice, a different kind of human being is created. Intuition increases, rapid healing responses occur, more thoughtful and aware personality traits are developed and the mind can become very subtle and keenly aware. Experiencing these higher human potentials can infuse our lives with a beauty that words can do little justice to. The world becomes safe again, your mind is no longer exhausted and fearful, the beauty of the natural world is more vibrant, and the burdens that we pile upon ourselves are lightened. Interfacing every day with the "open state" allows us to rest in this larger feeling, where the cares of this earth rest in the healing balm of Oneness.

MEDITATION AND STILLNESS

Hitting the relaxation response, trusting and surrendering to it might take some time. There may be a journey ahead of you. As you sit still, the parts of yourself that you might rather strangle and ignore could resurface. Sitting with the parts of yourself that you sent into exile may at first be uncomfortable. Years of resisting may have created a sort of festering way down deep inside. Drowning those painful memories and events with external short term gratification, and chaotic living generally does not offer a cure. The cure simply cannot occur until you are able to sit with the sensation long enough for the waves to crash upon the shores of your heart and mind and pass away on their own. There are many support systems out there to help you. A well trained psychologist, a spiritual councilor or support group may be in order for you. For some people, body centered psychotherapy works, like The Hakomi Method. For others groups like Alanon and AA might be more appropriate. If the sensations that arise produce unbearable emotional pain, it is time to reach out for support and help. Summon your courage, resiliency, and inner hero and do your best, little by little to sit with sensation until it resolves. In this way, you become adept at riding the waves of life with less desperation and more allowing acceptance of what is really true. You may find that the truth is just another bit of information, not good, not bad, but just what is. This will be an ongoing exploration until the very end of your days but in time, the journey may come to be interesting, fascinating, and note worthy instead of fearful, depressing and stressful. One of the best books I have ever read on understanding these concepts is *The Untetherd Soul* by Michael Singer. Within those pages Michael Singer describes the nature of the mind and the way we create our own insanity. His words are a pure transmission of a very high level of wisdom. Read it if you dare and meet yourself in the dark and private places within your own mind that have led you astray and caused great suffering. You will then find his gentle and yet laser sharp advice about how to gain freedom from the madness of this world and your own mind.

Chapter Highlights and Suggestions

Calming the central nervous system turns on our innate healing capacities. It returns the body to its natural state of rest and restoration. Focus, concentration, patience, and creativity are but a few of the benefits of a regular meditation practice. Begin today!

- There are many different kinds of meditation, try a few and find the ones that work best for you, there is no wrong way to meditate—except of course not meditating at all.

- Start small and build. 3-5 minutes a day is a wonderful start!

- Be sure your body is comfortable, use back, and knee support if needed.

- Use a guided meditation to start. Try calm.com. The basic version is free and very useful. Or try buddhify.com for more guided meditations.

- Begin by consciously relaxing your muscles and following your breath.

- If your mind wanders, worry not! Go back to your breath, or a word such as "peace" or "relax" or "stay."

- Focus on your body not your endless thoughts. Keep relaxing your muscles. Count your breath, that should keep you busy. Your mind will begin to get calm once your body remembers what it feels like to relax.

- Try a meditation group.

- Do your research. Books, classes, retreats, groups etc...get support and stay inspired.

- Meditation is just one part of the tapestry of life affirming practices.

- Movement and stillness are perfect compliments to each other. A regular movement practice will make your meditation practice easier as your spine will be stronger, more flexible and willing to stay still with more ease. A stiff, painful body will make sitting more challenging.

- Reach out for help if you feel despair or unbearable emotion surfacing as you get deeper into a meditative practice.

Reading and Audio List
(This is just a start! There are thousands of great books and audio out there):

Passionate Presence: Seven Qualities of Awakened Awareness by Catherine Ingram

Guided Meditation Series by Jon Kabat-Zinn (audio book)

Mindfulness for Beginners by Jon Kabat-Zinn (audio book)

The Minds Own Physician by Jon Kabat-Zinn (with The Dalai Lama and Richard Davidson)

Full Catastrophe Living (Revised Edition) by Jon Kabat-Zinn

The Emotional Life of Your Brain by Richard Davidson

The Miracle of Mindfulness by Thich Nhat Hahn

Fear: Essential Wisdom for Getting Through the Storm by Thich Nhat Hahn (audio book)

Emotional Awareness by The Dalai Lama

Waking Up in Time: Finding Inner Peace in Times of Accelerating Change by Peter Russell

A New Earth by Eckhart Tolle

The Untethered Soul by Michael Singer

The Medicine of the Future

In the future (or right now if you choose it) everyday medicine may not include a trip to the doctor or pharmacy. Instead each of us will be endowed with all the information we need to not only eradicate many common illnesses but if they should arise, we will know just what to do to bring ourselves back to health, sans the doctor or pharmacist.

In the past decade we've seen a steep rise in conditions that I'd like to call 'Lifestyle Disease'. Lifestyle Disease could be categorized as any condition that is brought on through repeated habits over time that alter the healthy function of the body. Illnesses like diabetes, heart disease, indigestion, gout, obesity, vascular disease and many more, could become rare if we heed the influx of scientific research and good old common sense currently making its way through our information highways. You are what you think, you are what you feel and you most surely are the result of what you do repeatedly over your life time. If you change your habits you change your cells, rapidly.

I predict that a time is fast approaching where the best doctors will be the ones that suggest you eat real food and move your body —without once touching the prescription pad. The best doctors will be the ones that encourage you to get up out of your office chair and have a brisk walk in the sunshine with a friend before enjoying a whole food lunch laden with fresh vegetables, lean protein and fresh clean water. Soda and fast food take-out? What soda and fast food take-out? One day we will see that those products are not for eating but for creating disease.

These doctors of the future will be few and far between because we will soon learn we can prescribe these medicines for ourselves. Our friends and family will remind us of the cure because everyone will simply understand the recipe for the needed lifestyle corrections. They will ask us: have you slept enough? Did you eat lots of vegetables today? Have you moved your body enough? Have you been outside enough? Did you paint, sing, dance or play this week? What have you been thinking about lately? If we get off track, we will be reminded of the things we need to do in order to restore ourselves to health.

We will still have use for doctors for things like broken bones, stitches, the occasional communicable disease, and research etc... but for the diseases of faulty lifestyle we will be responsible only to ourselves for the cure. Am I dreaming? Or will we, the people of this earth, finally grasp that we hold the key to our own vibrant health?

I for one, am rooting for us to turn towards The Medicine of the Future through the Human Restoration Project.

May you be happy, may you be peaceful and may your thoughts be gentle, beautiful and kind to yourself and all other beings.

For more info please visit:

www.outskirtspress.com/TheHumanRestorationProject
www.dynamicstillpoint.com
http://thehumanrestorationproject.blogspot.com

CPSIA information can be obtained at www.ICGtesting.com
Printed in the USA
BVOW11s0828110614

356063BV00011B/799/P